CFRN
Exam

SECRETS

Study Guide
Your Key to Exam Success

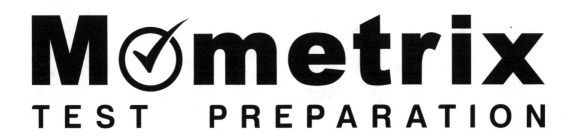

DEAR FUTURE EXAM SUCCESS STORY

First of all, **THANK YOU** for purchasing Mometrix study materials!

Second, congratulations! You are one of the few determined test-takers who are committed to doing whatever it takes to excel on your exam. **You have come to the right place.** We developed these study materials with one goal in mind: to deliver you the information you need in a format that's concise and easy to use.

In addition to optimizing your guide for the content of the test, we've outlined our recommended steps for breaking down the preparation process into small, attainable goals so you can make sure you stay on track.

We've also analyzed the entire test-taking process, identifying the most common pitfalls and showing how you can overcome them and be ready for any curveball the test throws you.

Standardized testing is one of the biggest obstacles on your road to success, which only increases the importance of doing well in the high-pressure, high-stakes environment of test day. Your results on this test could have a significant impact on your future, and this guide provides the information and practical advice to help you achieve your full potential on test day.

Your success is our success

We would love to hear from you! If you would like to share the story of your exam success or if you have any questions or comments in regard to our products, please contact us at **800-673-8175** or **support@mometrix.com**.

Thanks again for your business and we wish you continued success!

Sincerely,
The Mometrix Test Preparation Team

> **Need more help? Check out our flashcards at:**
> **http://MometrixFlashcards.com/CFRN**

TABLE OF CONTENTS

Introduction

Thank you for purchasing this resource! You have made the choice to prepare yourself for a test that could have a huge impact on your future, and this guide is designed to help you be fully ready for test day. Obviously, it's important to have a solid understanding of the test material, but you also need to be prepared for the unique environment and stressors of the test, so that you can perform to the best of your abilities.

For this purpose, the first section that appears in this guide is the **Secret Keys**. We've devoted countless hours to meticulously researching what works and what doesn't, and we've boiled down our findings to the five most impactful steps you can take to improve your performance on the test. We start at the beginning with study planning and move through the preparation process, all the way to the testing strategies that will help you get the most out of what you know when you're finally sitting in front of the test.

We recommend that you start preparing for your test as far in advance as possible. However, if you've bought this guide as a last-minute study resource and only have a few days before your test, we recommend that you skip over the first two Secret Keys since they address a long-term study plan.

If you struggle with **test anxiety**, we strongly encourage you to check out our recommendations for how you can overcome it. Test anxiety is a formidable foe, but it can be beaten, and we want to make sure you have the tools you need to defeat it.

Secret Key #1 – Plan Big, Study Small

There's a lot riding on your performance. If you want to ace this test, you're going to need to keep your skills sharp and the material fresh in your mind. You need a plan that lets you review everything you need to know while still fitting in your schedule. We'll break this strategy down into three categories.

Information Organization

Start with the information you already have: the official test outline. From this, you can make a complete list of all the concepts you need to cover before the test. Organize these concepts into groups that can be studied together, and create a list of any related vocabulary you need to learn so you can brush up on any difficult terms. You'll want to keep this vocabulary list handy once you actually start studying since you may need to add to it along the way.

Time Management

Once you have your set of study concepts, decide how to spread them out over the time you have left before the test. Break your study plan into small, clear goals so you have a manageable task for each day and know exactly what you're doing. Then just focus on one small step at a time. When you manage your time this way, you don't need to spend hours at a time studying. Studying a small block of content for a short period each day helps you retain information better and avoid stressing over how much you have left to do. You can relax knowing that you have a plan to cover everything in time. In order for this strategy to be effective though, you have to start studying early and stick to your schedule. Avoid the exhaustion and futility that comes from last-minute cramming!

Study Environment

The environment you study in has a big impact on your learning. Studying in a coffee shop, while probably more enjoyable, is not likely to be as fruitful as studying in a quiet room. It's important to keep distractions to a minimum. You're only planning to study for a short block of time, so make the most of it. Don't pause to check your phone or get up to find a snack. It's also important to **avoid multitasking**. Research has consistently shown that multitasking will make your studying dramatically less effective. Your study area should also be comfortable and well-lit so you don't have the distraction of straining your eyes or sitting on an uncomfortable chair.

The time of day you study is also important. You want to be rested and alert. Don't wait until just before bedtime. Study when you'll be most likely to comprehend and remember. Even better, if you know what time of day your test will be, set that time aside for study. That way your brain will be used to working on that subject at that specific time and you'll have a better chance of recalling information.

Finally, it can be helpful to team up with others who are studying for the same test. Your actual studying should be done in as isolated an environment as possible, but the work of organizing the information and setting up the study plan can be divided up. In between study sessions, you can discuss with your teammates the concepts that you're all studying and quiz each other on the details. Just be sure that your teammates are as serious about the test as you are. If you find that your study time is being replaced with social time, you might need to find a new team.

Secret Key #2 – Make Your Studying Count

You're devoting a lot of time and effort to preparing for this test, so you want to be absolutely certain it will pay off. This means doing more than just reading the content and hoping you can remember it on test day. It's important to make every minute of study count. There are two main areas you can focus on to make your studying count:

Retention

It doesn't matter how much time you study if you can't remember the material. You need to make sure you are retaining the concepts. To check your retention of the information you're learning, try recalling it at later times with minimal prompting. Try carrying around flashcards and glance at one or two from time to time or ask a friend who's also studying for the test to quiz you.

To enhance your retention, look for ways to put the information into practice so that you can apply it rather than simply recalling it. If you're using the information in practical ways, it will be much easier to remember. Similarly, it helps to solidify a concept in your mind if you're not only reading it to yourself but also explaining it to someone else. Ask a friend to let you teach them about a concept you're a little shaky on (or speak aloud to an imaginary audience if necessary). As you try to summarize, define, give examples, and answer your friend's questions, you'll understand the concepts better and they will stay with you longer. Finally, step back for a big picture view and ask yourself how each piece of information fits with the whole subject. When you link the different concepts together and see them working together as a whole, it's easier to remember the individual components.

Finally, practice showing your work on any multi-step problems, even if you're just studying. Writing out each step you take to solve a problem will help solidify the process in your mind, and you'll be more likely to remember it during the test.

Modality

Modality simply refers to the means or method by which you study. Choosing a study modality that fits your own individual learning style is crucial. No two people learn best in exactly the same way, so it's important to know your strengths and use them to your advantage.

For example, if you learn best by visualization, focus on visualizing a concept in your mind and draw an image or a diagram. Try color-coding your notes, illustrating them, or creating symbols that will trigger your mind to recall a learned concept. If you learn best by hearing or discussing information, find a study partner who learns the same way or read aloud to yourself. Think about how to put the information in your own words. Imagine that you are giving a lecture on the topic and record yourself so you can listen to it later.

For any learning style, flashcards can be helpful. Organize the information so you can take advantage of spare moments to review. Underline key words or phrases. Use different colors for different categories. Mnemonic devices (such as creating a short list in which every item starts with the same letter) can also help with retention. Find what works best for you and use it to store the information in your mind most effectively and easily.

3

Secret Key #3 – Practice the Right Way

Your success on test day depends not only on how many hours you put into preparing, but also on whether you prepared the right way. It's good to check along the way to see if your studying is paying off. One of the most effective ways to do this is by taking practice tests to evaluate your progress. Practice tests are useful because they show exactly where you need to improve. Every time you take a practice test, pay special attention to these three groups of questions:

- The questions you got wrong
- The questions you had to guess on, even if you guessed right
- The questions you found difficult or slow to work through

This will show you exactly what your weak areas are, and where you need to devote more study time. Ask yourself why each of these questions gave you trouble. Was it because you didn't understand the material? Was it because you didn't remember the vocabulary? Do you need more repetitions on this type of question to build speed and confidence? Dig into those questions and figure out how you can strengthen your weak areas as you go back to review the material.

Additionally, many practice tests have a section explaining the answer choices. It can be tempting to read the explanation and think that you now have a good understanding of the concept. However, an explanation likely only covers part of the question's broader context. Even if the explanation makes sense, **go back and investigate** every concept related to the question until you're positive you have a thorough understanding.

As you go along, keep in mind that the practice test is just that: practice. Memorizing these questions and answers will not be very helpful on the actual test because it is unlikely to have any of the same exact questions. If you only know the right answers to the sample questions, you won't be prepared for the real thing. **Study the concepts** until you understand them fully, and then you'll be able to answer any question that shows up on the test.

It's important to wait on the practice tests until you're ready. If you take a test on your first day of study, you may be overwhelmed by the amount of material covered and how much you need to learn. Work up to it gradually.

On test day, you'll need to be prepared for answering questions, managing your time, and using the test-taking strategies you've learned. It's a lot to balance, like a mental marathon that will have a big impact on your future. Like training for a marathon, you'll need to start slowly and work your way up. When test day arrives, you'll be ready.

Start with the strategies you've read in the first two Secret Keys—plan your course and study in the way that works best for you. If you have time, consider using multiple study resources to get different approaches to the same concepts. It can be helpful to see difficult concepts from more than one angle. Then find a good source for practice tests. Many times, the test website will suggest potential study resources or provide sample tests.

4

Practice Test Strategy

If you're able to find at least three practice tests, we recommend this strategy:

1. Take the first test with no time constraints and with your notes and study guide handy. Take your time and focus on applying the strategies you've learned.
2. Take the second practice test open-book as well, but set a timer and practice pacing yourself to finish in time.
3. Take any other practice tests as if it were test day. Set a timer and put away your study materials. Sit at a table or desk in a quiet room, imagine yourself at the testing center, and answer questions as quickly and accurately as possible.
4. Keep repeating step 3 on a regular basis until you run out of practice tests or it's time for the actual test. Your mind will be ready for the schedule and stress of test day, and you'll be able to focus on recalling the material you've learned.

Secret Key #4 – Pace Yourself

Once you're fully prepared for the material on the test, your biggest challenge on test day will be managing your time. Just knowing that the clock is ticking can make you panic even if you have plenty of time left. Work on pacing yourself so you can build confidence against the time constraints of the exam. Pacing is a difficult skill to master, especially in a high-pressure environment, so **practice is vital**.

Set time expectations for your pace based on how much time is available. For example, if a section has 60 questions and the time limit is 30 minutes, you know you have to average 30 seconds or less per question in order to answer them all. Although 30 seconds is the hard limit, set 25 seconds per question as your goal, so you reserve extra time to spend on harder questions. When you budget extra time for the harder questions, you no longer have any reason to stress when those questions take longer to answer.

Don't let this time expectation distract you from working through the test at a calm, steady pace, but keep it in mind so you don't spend too much time on any one question. Recognize that taking extra time on one question you don't understand may keep you from answering two that you do understand later in the test. If your time limit for a question is up and you're still not sure of the answer, mark it and move on, and come back to it later if the time and the test format allow. If the testing format doesn't allow you to return to earlier questions, just make an educated guess; then put it out of your mind and move on.

On the easier questions, be careful not to rush. It may seem wise to hurry through them so you have more time for the challenging ones, but it's not worth missing one if you know the concept and just didn't take the time to read the question fully. Work efficiently but make sure you understand the question and have looked at all of the answer choices, since more than one may seem right at first.

Even if you're paying attention to the time, you may find yourself a little behind at some point. You should speed up to get back on track, but do so wisely. Don't panic; just take a few seconds less on each question until you're caught up. Don't guess without thinking, but do look through the answer choices and eliminate any you know are wrong. If you can get down to two choices, it is often worthwhile to guess from those. Once you've chosen an answer, move on and don't dwell on any that you skipped or had to hurry through. If a question was taking too long, chances are it was one of the harder ones, so you weren't as likely to get it right anyway.

On the other hand, if you find yourself getting ahead of schedule, it may be beneficial to slow down a little. The more quickly you work, the more likely you are to make a careless mistake that will affect your score. You've budgeted time for each question, so don't be afraid to spend that time. Practice an efficient but careful pace to get the most out of the time you have.

6

Secret Key #5 – Have a Plan for Guessing

When you're taking the test, you may find yourself stuck on a question. Some of the answer choices seem better than others, but you don't see the one answer choice that is obviously correct. What do you do?

The scenario described above is very common, yet most test takers have not effectively prepared for it. Developing and practicing a plan for guessing may be one of the single most effective uses of your time as you get ready for the exam.

In developing your plan for guessing, there are three questions to address:

- When should you start the guessing process?
- How should you narrow down the choices?
- Which answer should you choose?

When to Start the Guessing Process

Unless your plan for guessing is to select C every time (which, despite its merits, is not what we recommend), you need to leave yourself enough time to apply your answer elimination strategies. Since you have a limited amount of time for each question, that means that if you're going to give yourself the best shot at guessing correctly, you have to decide quickly whether or not you will guess.

Of course, the best-case scenario is that you don't have to guess at all, so first, see if you can answer the question based on your knowledge of the subject and basic reasoning skills. Focus on the key words in the question and try to jog your memory of related topics. Give yourself a chance to bring the knowledge to mind, but once you realize that you don't have (or you can't access) the knowledge you need to answer the question, it's time to start the guessing process.

It's almost always better to start the guessing process too early than too late. It only takes a few seconds to remember something and answer the question from knowledge. Carefully eliminating wrong answer choices takes longer. Plus, going through the process of eliminating answer choices can actually help jog your memory.

Summary: Start the guessing process as soon as you decide that you can't answer the question based on your knowledge.

How to Narrow Down the Choices

The next chapter in this book (**Test-Taking Strategies**) includes a wide range of strategies for how to approach questions and how to look for answer choices to eliminate. You will definitely want to read those carefully, practice them, and figure out which ones work best for you. Here though, we're going to address a mindset rather than a particular strategy.

Your chances of guessing an answer correctly depend on how many options you are choosing from.

How many choices you have	How likely you are to guess correctly
5	20%
4	25%
3	33%
2	50%
1	100%

You can see from this chart just how valuable it is to be able to eliminate incorrect answers and make an educated guess, but there are two things that many test takers do that cause them to miss out on the benefits of guessing:

- Accidentally eliminating the correct answer
- Selecting an answer based on an impression

We'll look at the first one here, and the second one in the next section.

To avoid accidentally eliminating the correct answer, we recommend a thought exercise called **the $5 challenge**. In this challenge, you only eliminate an answer choice from contention if you are willing to bet $5 on it being wrong. Why $5? Five dollars is a small but not insignificant amount of money. It's an amount you could afford to lose but wouldn't want to throw away. And while losing $5 once might not hurt too much, doing it twenty times will set you back $100. In the same way, each small decision you make—eliminating a choice here, guessing on a question there—won't by itself impact your score very much, but when you put them all together, they can make a big difference. By holding each answer choice elimination decision to a higher standard, you can reduce the risk of accidentally eliminating the correct answer.

The $5 challenge can also be applied in a positive sense: If you are willing to bet $5 that an answer choice *is* correct, go ahead and mark it as correct.

Summary: Only eliminate an answer choice if you are willing to bet $5 that it is wrong.

8

Which Answer to Choose

You're taking the test. You've run into a hard question and decided you'll have to guess. You've eliminated all the answer choices you're willing to bet $5 on. Now you have to pick an answer. Why do we even need to talk about this? Why can't you just pick whichever one you feel like when the time comes?

The answer to these questions is that if you don't come into the test with a plan, you'll rely on your impression to select an answer choice, and if you do that, you risk falling into a trap. The test writers know that everyone who takes their test will be guessing on some of the questions, so they intentionally write wrong answer choices to seem plausible. You still have to pick an answer though, and if the wrong answer choices are designed to look right, how can you ever be sure that you're not falling for their trap? The best solution we've found to this dilemma is to take the decision out of your hands entirely. Here is the process we recommend:

Once you've eliminated any choices that you are confident (willing to bet $5) are wrong, select the first remaining choice as your answer.

Whether you choose to select the first remaining choice, the second, or the last, the important thing is that you use some preselected standard. Using this approach guarantees that you will not be enticed into selecting an answer choice that looks right, because you are not basing your decision on how the answer choices look.

This is not meant to make you question your knowledge. Instead, it is to help you recognize the difference between your knowledge and your impressions. There's a huge difference between thinking an answer is right because of what you know, and thinking an answer is right because it looks or sounds like it should be right.

Summary: To ensure that your selection is appropriately random, make a predetermined selection from among all answer choices you have not eliminated.

9

Test-Taking Strategies

This section contains a list of test-taking strategies that you may find helpful as you work through the test. By taking what you know and applying logical thought, you can maximize your chances of answering any question correctly!

It is very important to realize that every question is different and every person is different: no single strategy will work on every question, and no single strategy will work for every person. That's why we've included all of them here, so you can try them out and determine which ones work best for different types of questions and which ones work best for you.

Question Strategies

READ CAREFULLY

Read the question and answer choices carefully. Don't miss the question because you misread the terms. You have plenty of time to read each question thoroughly and make sure you understand what is being asked. Yet a happy medium must be attained, so don't waste too much time. You must read carefully, but efficiently.

CONTEXTUAL CLUES

Look for contextual clues. If the question includes a word you are not familiar with, look at the immediate context for some indication of what the word might mean. Contextual clues can often give you all the information you need to decipher the meaning of an unfamiliar word. Even if you can't determine the meaning, you may be able to narrow down the possibilities enough to make a solid guess at the answer to the question.

PREFIXES

If you're having trouble with a word in the question or answer choices, try dissecting it. Take advantage of every clue that the word might include. Prefixes and suffixes can be a huge help. Usually they allow you to determine a basic meaning. Pre- means before, post- means after, pro - is positive, de- is negative. From prefixes and suffixes, you can get an idea of the general meaning of the word and try to put it into context.

HEDGE WORDS

Watch out for critical hedge words, such as *likely, may, can, sometimes, often, almost, mostly, usually, generally, rarely,* and *sometimes.* Question writers insert these hedge phrases to cover every possibility. Often an answer choice will be wrong simply because it leaves no room for exception. Be on guard for answer choices that have definitive words such as *exactly* and *always.*

SWITCHBACK WORDS

Stay alert for *switchbacks.* These are the words and phrases frequently used to alert you to shifts in thought. The most common switchback words are *but, although,* and *however.* Others include *nevertheless, on the other hand, even though, while, in spite of, despite, regardless of.* Switchback words are important to catch because they can change the direction of the question or an answer choice.

10

FACE VALUE

When in doubt, use common sense. Accept the situation in the problem at face value. Don't read too much into it. These problems will not require you to make wild assumptions. If you have to go beyond creativity and warp time or space in order to have an answer choice fit the question, then you should move on and consider the other answer choices. These are normal problems rooted in reality. The applicable relationship or explanation may not be readily apparent, but it is there for you to figure out. Use your common sense to interpret anything that isn't clear.

Answer Choice Strategies

ANSWER SELECTION

The most thorough way to pick an answer choice is to identify and eliminate wrong answers until only one is left, then confirm it is the correct answer. Sometimes an answer choice may immediately seem right, but be careful. The test writers will usually put more than one reasonable answer choice on each question, so take a second to read all of them and make sure that the other choices are not equally obvious. As long as you have time left, it is better to read every answer choice than to pick the first one that looks right without checking the others.

ANSWER CHOICE FAMILIES

An answer choice family consists of two (in rare cases, three) answer choices that are very similar in construction and cannot all be true at the same time. If you see two answer choices that are direct opposites or parallels, one of them is usually the correct answer. For instance, if one answer choice says that quantity x increases and another either says that quantity x decreases (opposite) or says that quantity y increases (parallel), then those answer choices would fall into the same family. An answer choice that doesn't match the construction of the answer choice family is more likely to be incorrect. Most questions will not have answer choice families, but when they do appear, you should be prepared to recognize them.

ELIMINATE ANSWERS

Eliminate answer choices as soon as you realize they are wrong, but make sure you consider all possibilities. If you are eliminating answer choices and realize that the last one you are left with is also wrong, don't panic. Start over and consider each choice again. There may be something you missed the first time that you will realize on the second pass.

AVOID FACT TRAPS

Don't be distracted by an answer choice that is factually true but doesn't answer the question. You are looking for the choice that answers the question. Stay focused on what the question is asking for so you don't accidentally pick an answer that is true but incorrect. Always go back to the question and make sure the answer choice you've selected actually answers the question and is not merely a true statement.

EXTREME STATEMENTS

In general, you should avoid answers that put forth extreme actions as standard practice or proclaim controversial ideas as established fact. An answer choice that states the "process should be used in certain situations, if…" is much more likely to be correct than one that states the "process should be discontinued completely." The first is a calm rational statement and doesn't even make a definitive, uncompromising stance, using a hedge word *if* to provide wiggle room, whereas the second choice is a radical idea and far more extreme.

BENCHMARK

As you read through the answer choices and you come across one that seems to answer the question well, mentally select that answer choice. This is not your final answer, but it's the one that will help you evaluate the other answer choices. The one that you selected is your benchmark or standard for judging each of the other answer choices. Every other answer choice must be compared to your benchmark. That choice is correct until proven otherwise by another answer choice beating it. If you find a better answer, then that one becomes your new benchmark. Once you've decided that no other choice answers the question as well as your benchmark, you have your final answer.

PREDICT THE ANSWER

Before you even start looking at the answer choices, it is often best to try to predict the answer. When you come up with the answer on your own, it is easier to avoid distractions and traps because you will know exactly what to look for. The right answer choice is unlikely to be word-for-word what you came up with, but it should be a close match. Even if you are confident that you have the right answer, you should still take the time to read each option before moving on.

General Strategies

TOUGH QUESTIONS

If you are stumped on a problem or it appears too hard or too difficult, don't waste time. Move on! Remember though, if you can quickly check for obviously incorrect answer choices, your chances of guessing correctly are greatly improved. Before you completely give up, at least try to knock out a couple of possible answers. Eliminate what you can and then guess at the remaining answer choices before moving on.

CHECK YOUR WORK

Since you will probably not know every term listed and the answer to every question, it is important that you get credit for the ones that you do know. Don't miss any questions through careless mistakes. If at all possible, try to take a second to look back over your answer selection and make sure you've selected the correct answer choice and haven't made a costly careless mistake (such as marking an answer choice that you didn't mean to mark). This quick double check should more than pay for itself in caught mistakes for the time it costs.

PACE YOURSELF

It's easy to be overwhelmed when you're looking at a page full of questions; your mind is confused and full of random thoughts, and the clock is ticking down faster than you would like. Calm down and maintain the pace that you have set for yourself. Especially as you get down to the last few minutes of the test, don't let the small numbers on the clock make you panic. As long as you are on track by monitoring your pace, you are guaranteed to have time for each question.

DON'T RUSH

It is very easy to make errors when you are in a hurry. Maintaining a fast pace in answering questions is pointless if it makes you miss questions that you would have gotten right otherwise. Test writers like to include distracting information and wrong answers that seem right. Taking a little extra time to avoid careless mistakes can make all the difference in your test score. Find a pace that allows you to be confident in the answers that you select.

KEEP MOVING

Panicking will not help you pass the test, so do your best to stay calm and keep moving. Taking deep breaths and going through the answer elimination steps you practiced can help to break through a stress barrier and keep your pace.

Final Notes

The combination of a solid foundation of content knowledge and the confidence that comes from practicing your plan for applying that knowledge is the key to maximizing your performance on test day. As your foundation of content knowledge is built up and strengthened, you'll find that the strategies included in this chapter become more and more effective in helping you quickly sift through the distractions and traps of the test to isolate the correct answer.

Now it's time to move on to the test content chapters of this book, but be sure to keep your goal in mind. As you read, think about how you will be able to apply this information on the test. If you've already seen sample questions for the test and you have an idea of the question format and style, try to come up with questions of your own that you can answer based on what you're reading. This will give you valuable practice applying your knowledge in the same ways you can expect to on test day.

Good luck and good studying!

14

General Principles of Transport Nursing Practice

CLASSIC STRESSES OF FLIGHT

Decreased partial pressure of oxygen is one of eight classic stresses of flight; this stress can impact how blood cells absorb and carry oxygen. Changes in barometric pressure that generally occur during ascent and descent can affect gases trapped in certain areas of a patient's body, which can cause uncomfortable expansion throughout areas such as the sinuses, middle ear, and lungs. Body temperature regulation difficulties can occur during flight, as increases in altitude result in decreases in surrounding temperatures. As a result, hyperthermia and hypothermia can occur, which can lead to further medical complications. Decreased humidity occurs at high altitudes, which can result in significant moisture loss throughout the aircraft. Consequently, measures need to be implemented during transport to prevent dehydration. Noise from various components of the transport environment, aircraft vibration, fatigue caused by operational responsibilities of transport, and forces of gravity are all classic flight stresses as well.

As altitude increases, barometric pressure decreases. This can lead to increased flow rates through tubings. When possible, use pumps to maintain specific flow rates. In line rate controllers can prevent increases in fluid rate, but doesn't prevent decreases. When possible, use soft IV bags, but if using a glass IV bottle is necessary, the bottle must be vented, should be wrapped in a heavy cloth and taped, and should be hung over the patient's feet area, not head, in case gas expansion at altitude shatters the bottle.

HYPOXIA

Hypoxia is a condition characterized by an oxygen deficit within a patient's body; there are four categories of the condition. Hypoxic hypoxia occurs when a reduced amount of oxygen enters a patient's blood. Causes include conditions that block alveolar exchange like pneumonia and decreased pressures of oxygen at altitude. Hypemic hypoxia occurs when the blood's ability to transport oxygen to the tissues throughout a patient's body is diminished. Causes include anemia, hemorrhage, CO poisoning, sickle cell. Stagnant hypoxia occurs when blood flow is not sufficient. Causes include vasodilation, venous pooling due to G-forces, CPAP, G-forces, heart failure and decreased blood volume. Patients with stagnant hypoxia generally have well-oxygenated blood; the flow of that blood is just impeded. Histotoxic hypoxia occurs when a patient's tissue is not able to utilize oxygen. With histotoxic hypoxia, the amount of oxygen reaching the tissue is sufficient; disabled enzymes just make it difficult for the tissue to properly use the oxygen. Causes include narcotics, alcohol, and cyanide poisoning.

Recognizing hypoxia and potential for hypoxia early is important in preventing further emergencies for the patient. Recognizing the specific cause of a patient's hypoxia leads to more rapid and specific intervention leading to improved outcomes.

STAGES

Air transport can lead to several changes in a patient's cardiovascular system. These changes can include hypoxia, which is a deficit of oxygen within a patient's body. The severity of the oxygen deficit can range. There are four major stages of hypoxia. In the indifferent/asymptomatic phase there are not many noticeable effects for a healthy body. The primary symptom is loss of night and color vision, which would be significant for pilots. During the compensatory stage, usually occurring

15

around 10,000 feet, the healthy body will compensate for the changes by increasing CO and rate and depth of respirations. During the disturbance/deterioration stage, even healthy people may not be able to compensate leading to SOB, diminished vision, drowsiness, difficulty thinking, and incoordination. During the critical stage, there is almost complete incapacitation. This can lead to loss of consciousness and death. Air medical associated hypoxia can be decreased by providing oxygen and flying at lower altitudes, but due to terrain and weather this can be challenging. There are tables to assist CFRNs in determining a patient's oxygen needs to maintain the O_2 saturation at different altitudes. For example, a patient who is on .50 FIO_2 at sea level will need to be on .63 FIO_2 at an altitude of 6,000 feet and .98 FIO_2 at 12,000 feet to maintain close to the same SpO_2 levels. Patients with COPD should be kept at SpO_2 levels that are normal for the patient.

HAPE

High-altitude pulmonary edema (HAPE) occurs when fluid accumulates in the lungs. Early symptoms of HAPE can include a dry cough and shortness of breath; oftentimes, the shortness of breath can occur after only mild activity. As HAPE progresses, patients often notice that they are short of breath even when they are not exerting themselves. Very severe cases of HAPE may be accompanied by signs of gasping for breath or making sounds similar to gurgling during breathing. HAPE can also affect mental functioning, as a common symptom is confusion. Additional symptoms of HAPE can include a low-grade fever, sputum tinged with blood, and/or cyanosis – particularly of the lips and fingernails – which is a condition characterized by a bluish skin tone.

HACE

High-altitude cerebral edema (HACE) occurs when a significant amount of fluid accumulates in the brain. Symptoms of HACE may start out mild, but the condition can cause rapid deterioration in patients and can turn into a life-threatening condition in a short period of time. Similar to high-altitude pulmonary edema (HAPE), HACE can also affect mental functioning, as a common symptom is confusion. Headaches are another common symptom of the condition. As brain functioning becomes more affected by the condition, HACE can result in an abnormal and unstable gait. If HACE progresses into a life-threatening condition, patients often enter into a comatose state.

VIOLENT PATIENTS
ASSESSING AND MANAGING BEHAVIOR

One of the most important aspects of dealing with a violent patient is to assess the situation. The assessment should be conducted in a private, secure environment, but it should not be isolated or limited in terms of space. Assessing a violent patient in an isolated, limited environment increases the opportunities for the patient to act aggressively toward the individual(s) performing the assessment. Identifying the root cause(s) of the violent behavior is essential to effectively managing and/or eliminating the behavior. Physical restraint is often necessary in situations involving violent patients; however, physical restraint must be delivered in a manner that minimizes the risk of causing further medical complications. Additionally, physical restraints should only be implemented in situations where a sufficient number of trained professionals are available to assist with the restraints. If physical restraints do not successfully manage the patient's violent behavior, chemical restraint may also be considered.

COMMUNICATION TECHNIQUES

When dealing with a violent patient, it is essential to always communicate in a calm tone and to deliver consistent messages. It is important for the healthcare professional who is dealing with the patient to convey a sense of control and authority over the situation. At the same time, the professional should communicate to the patient that he/she will not be harmed in the current environment. Offering empathy to the patient about his/her feelings can be an effective strategy for minimizing aggression. Another effective communication strategy is to validate the patient's feelings rather than minimize them; in doing so, however, it is imperative that the professional does not validate the patient's violent behavior. Setting limits and clearly outlining consequences of violent behavior may help minimize the behavior as well. Additionally, the healthcare professional may communicate alternatives to the patient for his/her aggression, alternatives such as expressing feelings openly.

PROPER PATIENT EXTRICATION

Extrication involves the removal of forces that are restricting a patient and/or holding him/her back from moving freely. When moving an object or force from a patient, the first step in the process is to remove items around the patient that are confining him/her in a limited space. During the extrication process, it is important to offer emotional support to the patient; one way to offer support is to describe what is being done during the process. Throughout the process, flight team members should always be cognizant of the patient's location in relation to removing other objects and/or forces and do everything possible to protect the patient's safety. Using special extrication equipment, the next step of the process involves generating new openings around the patient and/or expanding openings that already exist in order to facilitate the final removal of the forces.

SITE REQUIREMENTS FOR NONDESIGNATED AIRCRAFT LANDING ZONE

A nondesignated landing zone (LZ) must be a size at least two times as large as the helicopter's length and width. An LZ 100 feet by 100 feet in size is a recommended guideline to follow; however, certain locations may have different requirements. The LZ must be a firm, smooth surface, and it must be as level a surface as possible in the given area. If possible, it is ideal for the LZ to be close to the patient; however, landing in close proximity to the patient is not essential if it jeopardizes the patient's safety or condition. The LZ – as well as the approach and departure path – should be free of any debris, wires, or other obstacles. An individual on the ground must be available to communicate with the pilot via radio regarding ground conditions such as wind and other potential hazards.

RISKS ASSOCIATED WITH ROTOR WASH

Rotor wash refers to the wind that is created by the rotor blades of a helicopter; rotor wash can produce winds greater than 50 miles per hour. The wind created by the rotor blades can cause dust, dirt, and debris to fly around, and it can cause loose articles of clothing, medical supplies, and any other unsecured items to blow way. Additionally, items at the scene that are not secured can potentially damage the engine of the helicopter if they become sucked into its air intake. Consequently, the flight team needs to ensure that all items at a transport scene are properly secured to minimize the risks of loss and engine damage. Furthermore, flight team members need to wear protective eyewear in order to minimize the risk of damaging their eyes from flying dust, dirt, and debris.

TYPES OF RADIO BANDS

The very high frequency (VHF) high-band frequency modulation (FM), which ranges from 148 to 174 megahertz (MHz), offers a straight line radio signal. The VHF low-band FM, which ranges from 30 to 50 MHz, has the greatest range, as it follows the Earth's curvature. With ranges from 118 to 136 MHz, the VHF amplitude modulation (AM) is generally the band used for radio communication related to aviation. Ultra-high frequency (UHF) radio bands, which range from 403 to 941 MHz, provide a limited range of communication; they are most effective when used between ground units and base stations. UHF radio bands can be used to communicate between the ground and the air, but only for short distances. Computer-controlled digital communication – 800 MHz – provides the ability for multiple organizations to communicate with one another. This radio band offers a higher frequency and less noise than others.

COMMONLY USED RESPONSE CODES FOR EMERGENCY VEHICLES RESPONDING TO CALLS

When an emergency vehicle responds to a call, the emergency medical personnel need to determine whether the transport status should be categorized as emergent or non-emergent. A code 1 – referred to as a cold response in certain agencies – indicates a non-emergent transport whereby no emergency lights or sirens should be used. When an emergency vehicle turns its lights on without utilizing the sirens, the response code is known as a code 2. A code 3 – referred to as a hot response in certain agencies – denotes a transport situation of emergent status whereby both emergency lights and sirens should be used.

SIMPLEX AND MULTIPLEX RADIO COMMUNICATION SYSTEMS

A simplex radio communication system is one in which communication can only occur in one direction at a time. For example, one party involved in the communication process can transmit a message to the receiving party. If both parties attempt to transmit messages simultaneously, one of the messages will be blocked. In contrast, a multiplex radio communication system is one in which two or more types of information can be transmitted simultaneously using the same radio frequency. For example, a multiplex system has the ability to transmit electrocardiogram (ECG) data via radio at the same time voice communication is being transmitted via radio.

PATIENT-RELATED INFORMATION OBTAINED BY FLIGHT TRANSPORT TEAM PRIOR TO TRANSPORT

Information gathered prior to transport is particularly important when the mode of transport is a fixed-wing aircraft, as flight times of such aircraft tend to be much longer than those of rotor-wing aircraft. Consequently, it is essential to gather an accurate description of the diagnosis and the current condition of the patient being transferred. Having correct information about the patient's diagnosis and medical status can assist the flight transport team in determining the most appropriate medical personnel and medical equipment to have available on the aircraft prior to transport. Additionally, the flight transport team should attempt to collect as much information as possible about who will accompany the patient on the flight as well as the weight of the patient, the weight(s) of the accompanying party or parties, and luggage weight. Finally, the transport team should ascertain whether the patient being transported has a "do not resuscitate" order in effect.

INFORMATION SUPPLIED WHEN PROVIDING UPDATED FLIGHT POSITION REPORTS

It is recommended that an updated flight position report be communicated every 15 minutes when an aircraft is within radio range. When communicating such reports, the flight team should be prepared to supply the identification number of the aircraft in addition to a general description of the aircraft. The general description should include information such as the model of the aircraft, the color of the aircraft, and how the aircraft is arranged. The current position of the aircraft as well as an estimated time of arrival to the destination should be supplied, and changes to the original flight plan route should be noted during the update reports.

PHYSICAL EXAMINATION FINDINGS REPORTED TO RECEIVING FACILITY

When reporting a patient's condition to a receiving facility, the first component of the physical examination that should be addressed is the patient's ABC status – the functioning of his/her airway, breathing, and circulation. The patient's neurological status should be reported to the receiving facility, and – if applicable – his/her Glasgow Coma Scale score should be provided as well. Abnormal findings encountered during a head-to-toe examination of the patient should be emphasized, and general findings from such an assessment should also be addressed. Additionally, the receiving facility should be informed of the patient's electrocardiogram (ECG) rhythm and his/her vital signs.

CREW RESOURCE MANAGEMENT

Crew resource management (CRM), also known as cockpit resource management, encompasses procedures designed to eliminate the risks associated with human error, which often results from inadequate leadership, ineffective teamwork, and poor decision-making. The focus of CRM is on interpersonal skills and improving communication among all crewmembers (rather than technical skills) to improve situational awareness which helps the crew better function as a team, carrying out problem solving and making decisions. CRM may include protocols for dealing with problems as well as checklists to ensure that no steps in a process are overlooked. While CRM was initially developed as part of aviation training, the basic procedures can be applied to virtually all aspects of healthcare. Classroom training is carried out in conjunction with flight simulation for all flight crewmembers. Topics include the information processing model, strategies to avoid human errors, workload over/underload, stress, fatigue, elements of situational awareness (perceiving, comprehending, and projecting), debriefing, coordinating, communicating, and automation.

TRANSPONDER CODES

A transponder code (AKA squawk code) is a unique code assigned to aircraft by air traffic controllers so that the aircraft can be identified on radar. Transponder codes contain 4 digits (0 through 7 only) transmitted by transponders with over 4096 different configurations possible. Directions for changing codes on dial models must be followed carefully to avoid accidentally signaling an emergency. Codes can be entered more easily on digital models. Aircraft on visual flight rules squawk 1200 in the United States when outside of controlled airspace but may be assigned a different code on entering controlled airspace.

In addition to the identifying code, emergency codes can be squawked.

- Emergency: 7700
- Radio failure: 7600
- Hijacking of aircraft: 7500

In addition to transponder codes, a pilot may use the term "Lifeguard" along with the aircraft call sign to indicate to air traffic controllers that the aircraft is an air ambulance flight and should have priority for assistance with facilitating flight.

GPS

The Global Positioning System (GPS) is a radio-navigation system operated by the US Air Force, based on satellite technology and utilized with mapping software to provide location information. GPS mapping software can provide address, location, and mapping directions for emergency medical services. GPS tracking devices to help locate places, individuals, and devices/equipment are increasingly present in smart phones, motor vehicles, aircraft, and even toys and shoes. GPS fleet tracking software can be utilized to track the location of a fleet of motor vehicles or aircraft in real time. GPS can also be utilized to determine the shortest route to a destination. However, mapping systems are not always up-to-date regarding changes (such as road closures), so errors can occur. Satellite signal interference may also cause problems, so ground crews should always have backup maps. GPS software should be routinely updated. The CFRN should be proficient in the use of local facility GPS and communication systems.

ELT

An emergency locator transmitter (ELT) is a tracking device that utilizes special frequencies to communicate emergency distress signals to satellites. The primary purpose of such a device is to track down individuals or groups in need of rescue in a timely manner in order to increase the chances of survival. In addition to distress signals, an ELT has the capacity to carry and transmit voice communication to search and rescue teams over an emergency frequency. Additionally, ELT units can be helpful in search and rescue efforts given that position and altitude can be communicated through the device. Considering the crucial nature of the first several hours following the occurrence of an injury or injuries, ELTs are vital components of any flight transport team.

NAVIGATION EQUIPMENT

The very-high frequency (VHF) Omni Range (VOR) offers pilots course guidance during non-precision approaches, which only utilize course information as opposed to course information plus slope and altitude information. While the VOR is the main aircraft radio navigation tool, it is starting to become obsolete as global positioning systems (GPS) are being utilized more frequently. The Distance Measuring Equipment (DME) communicates with the VOR by providing information about distance, ground speed, and time. The Instrument Landing System (ILS) is utilized during precision approaches at airports; it is the navigation tool most commonly used for such approaches. The ILS offers the pilot slope, altitude, and course runway guidance.

AIR MEDICAL RESOURCE MANAGEMENT

Air medical resource management is training for air medical professionals that includes flight and patient safety information with the goal of instituting a culture of safety. The focus is on the team building and strategies to facilitate a group working together and coping with changes. Air medical resource management includes all of the elements and procedures of crew resource management (including situational awareness, communication skills, workload issues, crew performance/coordination, and problem solving) but expands to include human factors (personality, group dynamics, behavior, physiology of flight, fatigue, and stress management) as well as resource management skills (use of checklists, dealing with automation, operating procedures). Training in risk management includes methods of mitigating risks that may occur and managing errors. According to the FAA, the four elements that must be included in air medical resource management training are (1) presentation skills (train-the-trainer), (2) initial indoctrination/awareness, (3) recurrent practice/feedback, and (4) continuing reinforcement.

NIGHT VISION GOGGLES

Night vision goggles are used for night flying by pilots and medical crewmembers to improve vision, especially in mountainous terrain and unimproved areas. NVGs comprise the mount (helmet), battery pack, and binocular assembly. The retina of the eye contains cone cells for daylight or high-intensity light vision (photopic vision) and rod cells for low intensity light vision (mesoptic [dawn, dusk, and moonlight]) vision or nighttime vision (scotopic vision). At night, color perception and fine details are lost, and a blind spot impairs central vision. Depth perception changes in low light, and image distortion occurs. Contrasts are often poor, such as between water and landmass; therefore, NVGs should only be utilized after appropriate training and individual fitting. Because exposure to bright lights impairs adaptation to the dark, crewmembers should wear sunglasses on the day of a night flight when outside, cockpit lighting should be dim blue-green, and uniforms and helmets should be dark. Techniques for NVGs include scanning from side to side, off-center viewing, and distance estimation.

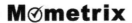

CIRCUMSTANCES UNDER WHICH FLIGHT TRANSPORT CREW SHOULD NOT SPEAK TO PILOT

While communication is an essential component of an effective air transport operation, there are certain times during the transport process when the flight team members should avoid communicating with the pilot unless the communication is deemed absolutely crucial. Two instances in which communication with the pilot should be avoided if it is not absolutely imperative are during takeoff and when the pilot is attempting to land the aircraft. Communication between the pilot and flight crew members should also be avoided, if possible, when the pilot is performing an instrument approach, which occurs when he/she attempts to land the aircraft in a situation of reduced visibility. Finally, when the pilot is navigating through areas of heavy air traffic, it is best for the flight team to refrain from engaging in non-essential communication with him/her.

AIRCRAFT SAFETY AT A LANDING SITE

While all members of the flight transport team are responsible for helping to maintain the safety of the aircraft, the pilot is ultimately responsible for aircraft security at a landing site. The pilot should be directed into the landing zone by a trained individual only. A ground-based incident commander should be in control of operations on the ground. While emergency personnel who are considered nonessential should remain 100 feet away from the landing zone, the incident commander should keep members of the general public at least 200 feet from the landing zone. Once the aircraft is on the ground, the pilot should be the only individual giving directions for patient care that takes place within the landing zone. Additionally, personnel should adhere to the pilot's instructions for approaching and departing the aircraft.

TYPES OF EMERGENCY LANDINGS

Land immediately refers to the notion that landing the aircraft is the top priority in order to make sure the individuals on board the aircraft survive. In this instance, the aircraft may land in an unsafe area not designated as a landing zone; however, unsafe landing areas such as trees or water should only be considered when no other landing option exists. Land as soon as possible means that the aircraft needs to land promptly but that a designated landing zone or appropriate landing site can be found prior to landing. In cases where the aircraft needs to land as soon as possible, unsafe landing areas should not be considered. Land as soon as practicable means that the pilot has the authority to determine an appropriate landing site and the length of the flight; however, pilots are discouraged from passing appropriate landing zones that are equipped to assist the aircraft.

SECURING EQUIPMENT AND PATIENTS DURING FLIGHT TRANSPORT AND HIGH ALTITUDE CONCERNS

Flight nurses are responsible for ensuring that medical equipment and devices are properly secured on the aircraft. It is essential that flight nurses evaluate the security of such items prior to every flight, as the flight team members and/or the patient may be injured if a piece of unsecured equipment becomes a projectile during transport. Additionally, to prevent injury to the patient, the flight nurse must ensure that the patient is properly restrained; proper restraint includes keeping the patient away from the pilot and the aircraft controls. Pediatric patients must be restrained during flight; it is not acceptable for a pediatric patient to be held during transport. As such, they must be restrained in an acceptable car seat that is attached to the aircraft stretcher. If physical restraints are required for a combative patient, they must be applied prior to transport. Policies specific to individual flight transport programs govern the use of physical restraints.

According to Boyle's law, at high altitude and decreased atmospheric pressure, gas volume expands, so an endotracheal tube or Foley catheter balloon filled with air may over-distend and burst; thus, normal saline should be used, especially for flights over 6000 feet although they must be monitored carefully as some expansion may still occur. This volume expansion may also affect injuries, such as

21

pneumothorax. A tension pneumothorax may occur rapidly as altitude increases. Intracranial pressure may increase in those with open skull fractures as air becomes trapped and expands.

EFFECTS OF WEATHER ON FLIGHTS

Weather should be constantly monitored both before and during flights to determine if a change in the flight plan is indicated. Weather concerns:

- Wind: Can both decrease and increase air speeds. High winds may result in dangerous turbulence that makes securing or treating a patient difficult. High crosswinds may be dangerous for takeoff and landing. Aircraft are routinely grounded with hurricane force winds.
- Rain: Usually poses few problems because aircraft should be supplied with means to keep the windshields clean of rain, such as windscreen wipes or high pressure air systems that blow water off the windshield.
- Ice/Snow: Runways must be cleared to enable takeoff and landing. Aircraft may require de-icing prior to takeoff.
- Fog/Poor visibility (sandstorm, dust storm, fire): May result in flight delays or grounding of aircraft. When visibility is less than one mile, the airport must follow Low Visibility Procedures (LVPs), which can include reducing the number of aircraft allowed to land or take off in order to decrease risk of accidents.

PRE-TRANSPORT EQUIPMENT AND SUPPLY CHECK

A pre-transport check consists of an assessment of the availability of equipment and medical supplies; this assessment should follow a standardized list of equipment and supplies. Equipment and/or supplies that bear expiration dates should have their expirations verified; if any items are past their expiration dates, they should be replaced. Medical equipment that is used in patient care processes should be examined to determine whether it is functioning properly. Prior to each transport encounter, equipment and supplies that are deemed necessary and/or deemed possibly necessary during the transport process should be identified, as certain items that may not be standard need to be acquired before departure. Oxygen and air quantities should be checked prior to transport as well in order to verify that the supply of both gases is sufficient.

PPE THE TRANSPORT TEAM MEMBERS CAN WEAR DURING TRANSPORT PROCESS

Flight specific personal protective equipment (PPE) may consist of helmets, fire-resistant clothing, protective footwear, and/or hearing protectors. Helmets may potentially protect transport team members against head injuries. To obtain the greatest benefit from a helmet, it must fit appropriately, be lightweight and comfortable, and its lining must absorb energy. Uniforms that are fire-resistant may protect the flight crew from dangerous skin exposure and tissue damage that can occur during fires resulting from an aircraft accident. Protective footwear such as boots can provide team members with protection from injuries such as punctures and cuts. Earplugs or earmuffs can be worn when transport encounters involve extreme levels of noise; such hearing protection may protect against hearing loss. Universal PPE should be in the appropriate size for an individual:

- Eye protectors: Should be worn with risk of splash or spray with body fluids or contact with debris. (Prescription glasses do not take the place of goggles.)
- Face shields: Provide protection for face, eyes, nose, and mouth. Preferred to goggles when there is risk of spray or splash of body fluids.

- Masks: Protect the nose and mouth from fluids and particles and should be fluid resistant, fit snugly, and have a flexible nosepiece.
- Respirators (such as N95, N100): Protect the nose, mouth, and airway passages exposed to hazardous or infectious aerosols, ng bacteria (TB, measles patients).

USES FOR AIRCRAFT SEATS, TIRES, AND WINGS IN POST-CRASH SITUATIONS

Following a crash, the seats of the aircraft can be used for many purposes. The seats can provide insulation in shelters, they can offer materials to make sleeping more feasible, they can supply many materials to start fires, and – depending on the color of the seats – they can supply materials to create various signals for search-and-rescue aircraft. The aircraft tires can be used to create black smoke, which can in turn be used to signal search-and-rescue aircraft. Adding rubber to a fire creates black smoke, which may provide greater contrast – and, subsequently, more chances of creating a successful signal – with certain crash site environments. The wings of the aircraft can be utilized as collection devices for rain water and dew, they can function as wind breakers, they can be used to support shelters, and they can provide shade from the sun.

ROLE OF CLOTHING IN SURVIVAL SITUATIONS

Clothing plays an essential role in a survival situation, as it may serve as the only shelter an individual has from the environment. As such, in cold-weather environments, an individual's clothing may be the only barrier he/she has against hypothermia. Warm-weather environments call for clothing that provides adequate sun protection; long-sleeve shirts and pants are ideal for such environments. Head and eye gear should also be worn for protection against warm-weather elements. The most appropriate, effective clothing for flight transport personnel is clothing that is both comfortable and practical. Clothing that fits tightly should be avoided, as it may affect circulation and restrict movement, which is not ideal in the flight transport setting. Clothing that offers appropriate ventilation provides the best means of adequately regulating heat as well. Layers are ideal for clothing in the flight transport setting, as they can be removed or added as needed.

POTENTIAL DANGERS OF NATURAL SHELTERS

While natural shelters can provide flight team members with protection from environmental factors, they can also pose dangers. Dead trees and dead tree limbs can pose a threat of injury if they fall during strong winds. Additionally, trees and rocks can have the potential to conduct lightning. In addition to the issue of lightning, flight team members also need to be aware of the potential for dangerous rock slides if they choose to seek shelter around rocks or rock formations. While caves and other areas that offer burrowing potential can provide a great deal of natural shelter from storms, cold climates, and additional environmental factors, they can also be home to potentially dangerous inhabitants such as bears and mountain lions. These dangers do not negate the benefits of natural shelters; they only serve as reminders to flight team members to use extra caution when seeking out such protective spaces.

USING WATER DURING SURVIVAL SITUATIONS

Water should be rationed to prolong whatever supply the flight transport team has in order to help maintain adequate hydration levels. Water should be boiled or purified with a water purification tablet prior to consumption. Failing to purify water can lead to bacterial gastrointestinal issues, which can result in diarrhea and/or vomiting, two causes of rapid dehydration. When a survival situation occurs in a snow-filled environment, it is best to melt the snow, as consuming the snow directly can lead to significant body heat loss. Additionally, water kept in cold weather environments should be kept in open, shallow containers; this can help prevent the liquid from expanding and rupturing the container. If the flight team has instant beverage packets such as hot

23

chocolate and/or instant soup packets aboard the aircraft, it is ideal to mix the packets with water to gain the benefits of combining a meal with liquid.

RULE OF THREES

The *rule of threes* identifies how long the average person can survive without various life necessities. According to the rule, an average person can survive without oxygen for about three minutes. In extreme weather conditions, an average person can live without shelter from such conditions for three hours. The average person can survive without water for three days; he/she can live without food for three weeks. Once medical issues and safety concerns have been handled, the *rule of threes* can help a flight team prioritize their duties in a survival situation. The rule establishes that the flight team should first either seek or build shelter; following the creation of some type of safe shelter, the flight team should build a fire and send out smoke signals for assistance.

SIGNALING SEARCH-AND-RESCUE AIRCRAFT IN POST-CRASH SITUATIONS
SMOKE, SIGNAL MIRRORS, AND FLARES

When used to signal search-and-rescue aircraft in a post-crash situation, smoke is typically considered the most effective signal method to use during the day. With the addition of certain substances, smoke can be created as either black smoke or white smoke. The choice of which color smoke to use to signal should be determined based on which color provides the greatest contrast with the environment around the crash site. A signal mirror can be used by creating reflections off of shiny metal objects or cans found at the crash site or available on the aircraft. Signal mirrors are most effective on overcast days, which offer the greatest opportunities to cast strong reflections. For nighttime, flares or a flashlight – which can both typically be found aboard the aircraft – can be used to signal search-and-rescue teams.

CLOTHING, WHISTLES, DYES, AND SIGNAL PANELS

During the daytime, brightly colored clothing can assist the search-and-rescue aircraft with finding the crash site. Certain materials aboard the aircraft may be bright enough to help identify the site as well. Whistles can be used when search-and-rescue efforts occur on the ground; they are particularly useful at night or when poor weather conditions exist, as search-and-rescue teams will likely need guidance towards the crash site in such circumstances. If the crash site is located near snow or water, dyes offer a useful material for signaling. Furthermore, signal panels can be laid in a geometric pattern to help clearly mark the crash site.

SURVIVAL RESOURCES IN POST-CRASH SITUATIONS

After a crash, the aircraft's battery can be used to power signal lights, to facilitate communication with search-and-rescue teams by powering communication devices, and to help start fires. The doors of the aircraft can be used in post-crash situations as shelter materials, as devices to help break the wind, and to create geometric patterns to form signal panels to help search-and-rescue aircraft identify the crash site. The aircraft's engine fuel can also be used to start fires, which can in turn be used as smoke to signal search-and-rescue teams.

OPEN-SEA SURVIVAL

When the aircraft is flying over water, all team members should wear personal flotation devices. They should also prepare for the aircraft to turn over upon impact, a factor that will affect their evacuation plan. When the flight team members are actually in the water, they can attempt to control the amount of heat they lose by assuming the heat escape lessening posture (HELP), which can be done by bringing the knees to the chest and wrapping the arms around the knees; the position is basically identical to the fetal position. HELP is only effective in helping individuals stay

24

afloat, however, if the individual is utilizing a personal flotation device. Heat loss can also be counteracted if the flight team members huddle together in the water. Exposed skin surfaces should be protected from the sun and from the salt in the water by being covered, when possible.

CLEANING SOLUTIONS USED FOR DECONTAMINATION PURPOSES

Bleach – in a 1:10 milliliter (ml) solution – can decontaminate items composed of plastic. If areas such as the transport vehicle floor and stretcher mattresses do not have any dirt or dried blood, they can be cleaned with a bleach solution as well. A drawback to using bleach is its ability to discolor fabrics on items such as stretcher mattresses. Alcohol can be highly effective at decontaminating areas; however, it is flammable and extremely drying if it comes into contact with skin. As with bleach solution, alcohol should be used only on surfaces that do not have any dirt or dried blood present. Glutaraldehyde – diluted with water – is effective at decontaminating items made of plastic or vinyl. One drawback to using glutaraldehyde is that its acidic nature can cause corrosion; as such, it should not be used around electronic equipment aboard the transport vehicle and/or on items containing stainless steel.

PROPER DISPOSAL OF BIOHAZARDOUS WASTE

Biohazard bags should be used to collect dry solid waste such as medical gloves worn when treating a patient with an infectious disease. Leak-proof biohazard bags can also be used to collect waste that contains blood or other bodily fluids. Puncture-resistant containers designated for sharp items should be used to collect "sharps" such as needles. Potentially contaminated fluids suctioned from patients during flight transport should be enclosed in sealed containers; unnecessary handling of such fluids should be avoided during transport, particularly if a risk of splashing exists. Biohazard bags, sharps containers, and sealed containers should be properly disposed of at the destination facility according to the facility's local disposal requirements.

TRIAGE

Triage is the process of sorting patients by prioritizing care, treatment, and transportation based on injury severity. One benefit of triage is that it provides prompt medical care to those patients whose lives or limbs are in jeopardy. Triage also directly affects the medical facilities that are available to care for victims of disasters; by sorting patients based on injury severity and identifying those with minor injuries, the burden placed on the receiving hospitals is lessened, as they are not attempting to provide care to patients with only minor injuries. In turn, this benefit affects patients with the most severe injuries by creating more hospital time and personnel to care for those with life-threatening injuries. Triage also helps alleviate some of the burden placed on receiving hospitals when a disaster occurs by distributing casualties among several hospitals rather than burdening only one hospital with all of the victims.

CLASSIFICATION SYSTEM FOR TRIAGING DISASTER VICTIMS

Victims of disasters are triaged according to their potential for survival absent extraordinary life-saving techniques; they are also triaged according to the severity of their injuries in relation to other victims of the same disaster. Disaster victims are generally classified as: 1) immediate care; 2) delayed care; 3) minor care; or 4) dead. A victim requiring immediate care is a victim whose life can be saved if advanced medical intervention is initiated within one hour. A victim classified as requiring delayed care is one whose condition is not life-threatening and whose condition will not decline if medical attention is not initiated within one hour. Victims requiring minor care are those whose injuries are not severe; they can generally receive care on an outpatient basis in an ambulatory setting, and the care does not need to be provided within a certain amount of time following the occurrence of a disaster.

ADVANCED TRAUMA LIFE SUPPORT PROTOCOL

The Advanced Trauma Life Support protocol steps include:

- Primary Survey
- Airway with C-spine control
- Breathing (assess oxygenation and ventilation and correct if needed including chest tubes)
- Circulation (assess for and stop bleeding), IVs, response, tissue perfusion
- Disability (GCS, pupils, prevent secondary brain injury)
- Exposure/environmental (assess temp and correct, remove clothing)
- Adjuncts (foley, g-tube, hemodynamics/resp monitoring, ABGs, labs, etc.)
- Secondary Survey
- History
- Complete Head to toe physical exam
- Definitive Treatment
- Ongoing Assessment

ASSESSMENT OF RESPIRATION, PULSE, AND CIRCULATION ACCORDING TO THE START PLAN

According to the Simple Triage and Rapid Treatment (START) approach, if a non-ambulatory disaster victim is not breathing, attempts should be made to restore his/her breathing; if attempts are unsuccessful, the victim should be labeled as deceased. If the victim is breathing, triage personnel should evaluate his/her respiratory rate. If the victim's respiratory rate is greater than 30, he/she should be identified as needing immediate care, as the increased rate may indicate impending shock. If the rate is less than 30, perfusion should be performed, and pulse and circulation should be evaluated during the perfusion process.

According to the Simple Triage and Rapid Treatment (START) approach, perfusion should be performed on a non-ambulatory disaster victim if the victim's respiratory rate is less than 30. Pulse and circulation should be assessed during perfusion. A victim with no pulse should be identified as needing immediate care. If a pulse is detected, consciousness level should be evaluated by asking the victim to follow commands. Victims who are able to follow simple commands should be identified as delayed care victims while those who are not able to follow commands should be identified as immediate care. Circulation is evaluated using a capillary refill test; victims whose refill times are greater than two seconds should be labeled as immediate care, and victims whose refill times are less than two seconds should be evaluated to determine level of consciousness using the simple command test.

TRAINING ASSISTANCE MADE AVAILABLE AS PART OF THE 1996 DEFENSE AGAINST WEAPONS OF MASS DESTRUCTION ACT'S EMERGENCY RESPONSE ASSISTANCE PROGRAM

The Emergency Response Assistance Program created through the Defense Against Weapons of Mass Destruction Act of 1996 provides training to emergency preparedness personnel from federal, state, and local agencies in how to operate and maintain equipment that serves various purposes. Emergency preparedness personnel learn how to operate equipment that has the capability to detect biological and chemical agents as well as nuclear radiation. Additionally, they are trained to use equipment that can monitor biological and chemical agents and radiation. The program provides emergency response personnel with training on equipment designed to protect the response team members as well as the general public. Furthermore, they receive training on equipment used for decontamination purposes.

EVALUATING WHETHER PUBLISHED EVIDENCE-BASED RESEARCH IS APPLICABLE TO CLINICAL PRACTICE

Evidence-based research refers to the development of clinical guidelines. Certain components of the research can be examined to determine its applicability to clinical practice. Looking at what experts conducted the research and what the skills and backgrounds of those experts are can offer insight about the credibility of the research. Two additional important components to look at are: 1) what framework the experts used to carry out their research; and 2) whether or not the clinical guideline has been tested. When reading published research studies, it is important to determine whether the sample size studied was sufficiently large to lead to the conclusions being drawn, whether the methods and instruments the researchers used to collect their data were valid and reliable, whether the research findings address a current clinical need, and whether the guidelines need to be evaluated further prior to implementation.

PRIMARY RULES OF HIPAA

The Health Insurance Portability and Accountability Act (HIPAA) covers three areas related to the protection of patient health information and to the transmission of claims made by healthcare providers. The first area is called the Transaction and Code Set Rule (TCS Rule); this rule set forth national standards by which all electronic healthcare transactions must adhere. To establish consistency, the TCS Rule also developed national identifiers for claims filed by healthcare providers. The TCS Rule does not have much of a direct impact on flight transport team members, as billing departments are typically responsible for electronic transactions. The second area – the Privacy Rule – established national standards for protecting patient health information and restricting access to protected health information (PHI). The final area is called the Security Rule, which sets forth national guidelines and protocols for healthcare organizations to follow in order to provide appropriate security against unwarranted access to PHI.

PHI

Protected health information (PHI) can be defined as any physical or mental health information that can be used to identify an individual. PHI can include information maintained in any type of record including oral accounts, written documentation, or electronic records. PHI includes information about the past, present, or future physical or mental health of an individual and/or records of care that patient received from a healthcare provider. PHI can also include demographic information about an individual that might render him/her easily identifiable. Finally, records of payment for services from an individual to a healthcare provider can also be considered PHI, as the conclusion can be drawn that the services being paid for provide information about the individual's past, present, or future physical or mental health.

EXCHANGING PHI WITHOUT PATIENT CONSENT UNDER THE TPO EXCEPTIONS

According to the Treatment, Payment, and Operations (TPO) exceptions, transport team members are able to disclose protected health information (PHI) to other individuals directly involved in the patient's care without first obtaining the patient's consent. Consequently, the transport team may discuss a patient's condition, status, past or present medical conditions, and the like with individuals at the scene, healthcare personnel at the receiving facility, and via radio transmissions without patient consent. The transport team may also exchange PHI for billing and payment purposes without obtaining consent. While the TPO exceptions place less restrictive guidelines on transport team members with regard to the exchange of PHI, the transport team is expected to disclose and receive the least amount of PHI necessary to meet the needs of the situation.

EMTALA COMPONENTS

The Emergency Medical Treatment and Active Labor Act (EMTALA) includes the following components:

- any patient who arrives at an emergency department and requests an examination to determine the presence or absence of an emergency medical condition shall be provided such an examination
- if an emergency medical condition is present, emergency department personnel are required to provide services to stabilize the patient or to arrange for the patient to be transferred to a different facility once he/she is stabilized
- if the patient must be transferred, the transfer facility must have the space and personnel necessary to care for the patient
- in the case of a transfer, the referring facility must provide all necessary documentation to the transfer site
- qualified personnel, necessary medical equipment, and the most appropriate transport mode must be available in the case of a patient transfer

INFORMED CONSENT

Informed consent involves obtaining consent to provide medical treatment to a patient once the patient has been informed of potential risks of the treatment as well as limitations of the treatment. If more than one treatment option is available to a patient, each option and its associated risks and limitations must be outlined for the patient prior to obtaining consent to treat. The fundamental premise of informed consent is that the patient fully comprehends what is being explained to him/her and that he/she subsequently has the competence to either consent to or refuse treatment based on that comprehension. Due to their age, minors are not able to provide informed consent for themselves and, therefore, must have a parent or legal guardian do so. Additionally, the patient must have all his/her faculties intact and be free from any sort of impairment at the time of consent.

EVALUATING WHETHER PATIENT IS CAPABLE OF OFFERING INFORMED CONSENT TO TREATMENT

A patient is capable of providing informed consent if his/her faculties are all intact and if the patient is not impaired in any capacity. A patient must be given a chance to provide his/her informed consent for treatment as long as he/she is conscious and coherent to the point of understanding the potential risks and limitations associated with each treatment option as they are presented by the flight transport team. Examples of patients who may not have all their faculties intact are patients who are mentally ill or intellectually disabled. Examples of patients who would not be able to provide informed consent due to impairment are individuals who are under the influence of alcohol or other drugs and individuals whose senses are weakened due to a medical condition, illness, or other health-related problem.

SIGNS OF ELDER ABUSE AND/OR NEGLECT

Common signs of elder abuse and/or neglect can include – but are not limited to – the following:

- medication overdoses, which can be confirmed through laboratory tests
- medical problems that have not been treated
- bruises and/or cuts that cannot be explained
- indications that the elder patient has been restrained in some way
- inability to easily move extremities due to muscle stiffness
- fractured bones

- indications that the elder patient is not bathed or clean
- bleeding in the vaginal or anal areas that cannot be explained may indicate sexual abuse

SIGNS OF CHILD ABUSE AND/OR NEGLECT

Common signs of child abuse and/or neglect can include – but are not limited to – the following:

- burns, bruises, or skin lacerations that may resemble the form of an object may indicate abuse
- children who are abused have a tendency to fear all adults, not just the adult(s) who is(are) abusing the child; alternatively, children who are sexually abused may express fear of a particular adult
- children who are abused may express a desire not to return to their homes
- anger, depression, and/or focus difficulties may signify emotional abuse
- an emaciated appearance and/or extreme hunger can indicate neglect
- indications that the child is not bathed or clean
- missing clumps or patches of hair

SIGNS OF DOMESTIC VIOLENCE

Common signs of domestic violence can include – but are not limited to – the following:

- injuries to the patient's head are common in domestic violence cases; such injuries may include broken teeth or fractured jaws, ear drum perforations, and/or broken noses
- bruising throughout the patient's body and/or bruising concentrated in one location on the patient's body
- bite marks determined to be caused by adult teeth
- indications that the patient has been strangled or choked may occur in domestic violence cases; such indications can include ligature marks on the neck, bruising and lacerations or finger marks about the neck, damage to the larynx, and neck vein distention

ACEP GUIDELINES FOR AMBULANCE DIVERSION

According to the American College of Emergency Physicians (ACEP), Emergency Medical Services (EMS) systems should develop policies that are mutually agreed upon by EMS systems and other agencies regarding diversion. The ACEP believes that such policies should be established to address certain objectives; those objectives include:

- identifying situations where temporary diversion may be required, particularly situations in which hospital resources such as personnel and beds are insufficient;
- designating a primary EMS agency or central communication facility to inform EMS teams and hospitals when a facility is on diversion
- evaluating the facility's diversion status in a regular manner and continuing to provide updates to affected EMS systems and other agencies
- implementing practices that allow for the safe, appropriate, and timely care of patients who enter the system during an active diversion period
- establishing procedures that lower the likelihood of diversions

INFORMATION INCLUDED IN DOCUMENTATION OF TRANSPORT CARE

Documentation should always include a log of the patient's complaints, the patient's symptoms related to his/her complaints, and the nurse's responses to each complaint. As a means of charting changes in the patient, this component of the documentation process should be recorded at regular intervals throughout transport. Detailed notes should be recorded about the patient's condition

29

prior to receiving treatment as well as response(s) to such treatment. Documentation that outlines the chain of care – including specific names of personnel as well as responsibilities of those individuals – should be provided. Medical histories and medications the patient is currently taking are also valuable pieces of information to document. Suspected drug or alcohol use should be documented; if the patient readily admits to drug or alcohol use, his/her comments should be documented directly and placed in quotes to signify that the comments are the patient's exact words.

DOCUMENTATION PROCESS WHEN CRITICAL INCIDENTS OCCUR DURING TRANSPORT

For critical incidents that occur either prior to or during transport, any details that are available about the incident should be documented. This should also include information about what was done in response to the incident and who was involved in the response. For critical incidents that occur prior to the patient being transported, documentation should include names of individuals who are able to provide information about the details of the incident, and the information those individuals provide should be documented in quotes to signify that the information is from someone other than the documenter. When critical incidents occur during transport, it is important to document a timeline of events including specific or approximate times. Documentation should also include information about what was done in response to the event and what procedures were followed during the response.

DIVERSITY PRACTICE MODEL

With respect to patient diversity, the Diversity Practice Model can help flight team members recognize what similarities and differences exist between them and their patients.

1. Assumption – flight team members should examine their assumptions about the individual and/or the community of which the individual is a member.
2. Beliefs or behaviors – flight team members should identify how their beliefs affect the type of care they provide and how they behave towards their patients.
3. Communication – the flight team should assess the patient's communication in terms of capability, language, and other senses such as sight and sound.
4. Diversity – visible factors, such as skin color and age, should be identified as possible areas of diversity, and factors that cannot be seen, such as socioeconomic status, should also be identified.
5. Education and Ethics – flight team members should learn what makes patients diverse and recognize that diversity affects ethical decisions.

CONFLICT RESOLUTION TECHNIQUES

It is important for all parties involved in conflict resolution to recognize that conflict is natural and normal and that it does not have to be destructive as long as the conflict is handled in an appropriate manner. Additionally, it is essential that all involved parties acknowledge that not everyone shares the same opinions and views about events and issues. For conflict resolution efforts to be successful, everyone involved must be willing to communicate effectively and to listen effectively; listening is just as important as – if not more important than – verbal communication during attempts to resolve conflicts. In order to ensure effective communication and to prevent misunderstandings, it is beneficial to summarize the other party's points and/or to clarify anything that is not clear. All parties involved should work together to come up with a solution to the conflict that is fair and beneficial to each of them.

COMMUNICATION WITH PATIENT'S FAMILY PRIOR TO TRANSPORT

As time permits and within the limitations of patient confidentiality, the transport team should communicate with the patient's family about what will be done to the patient during transport. In addition to discussing patient care with the family prior to transport, the family should be made aware of the logistics surrounding the transport. They should be informed of approximately how long the flight will last, and, if possible, they should be provided with driving directions to the facility where the patient is being transported. It is helpful to explain to the family where they should go upon arriving at the facility as well as how they should locate the transport team and/or the patient once they arrive. Depending on time, family concerns about the patient and his/her condition and/or about the transport procedures should be addressed before the transport team departs with the patient.

HANDLING RESPONSES OF ANGER, HOSTILITY, AND/OR DISTRUST FROM PATIENTS' FAMILIES

When a patient's family responds to a crisis with anger, hostility, and/or distrust, the transport team should provide the family with opportunities to voice their feelings. The root cause(s) behind the feelings must be identified in order to develop appropriate responses. It is important to let the family know that their feelings are normal and acceptable. Particularly in cases where a family expresses a lack of trust in the situation, it is important to implement a schedule of updates for the patient's family. Organized, regular updates about the patient may demonstrate the level of professionalism with which the team is handling the situation; ideally, family updates should be provided by the same individual(s) each time, as this can increase the family's level of trust and comfort. Team members can also talk with families about ways to turn their anger into positive energy that may benefit the patient and/or the situation.

SUPPORTING FAMILY MEMBERS FOLLOWING A PATIENT DEATH

Many people cope with death best by having the ability to see their loved one, which is why it may be beneficial for family members to view the patient's body at the scene. Following the death of a transport patient, many family members have a lot of questions; it is important that the transport team or additional healthcare professionals take the time to address all questions posed by the family. While some families have a lot of questions at the time of death, many do not think of their questions until after they have processed the death. Consequently, it is essential that the family understands how and why the patient's death occurred and that the patient received the highest level of clinical care possible. In every situation, compassion and professionalism should be exercised when responding to family members.

CQI AND QA

Continuous quality improvement (CQI) environments are very patient-centered, which is consistent with the direction health care in general has gone. Patients tend to be more involved in many aspects of their health care than they once were many years ago, and CQI programs support the role of the patient and the patient's family. Conversely, quality assurance (QA) programs operate based on a need to meet requirements that are externally mandated by organizations, laws/regulations, and/or agencies. Consequently, while QA activities are performed solely to serve the purpose of fulfilling a particular requirement, CQI environments are not hindered by such requirements, which allows them to focus solely on the needs of patients.

Quality assurance (QA) methodology has traditionally involved the use of evidence that cannot necessarily be supported and data from studies that have been conducted after the fact with little or no structure to them. Conversely, continuous quality improvement (CQI) programs rely on hard, verifiable data rather than opinions or feelings. Unlike QA environments, CQI environments employ a standardized formula for solving problems rather than solving problems and making decisions using a method that does not lead to predictable results.

CLINICAL AND LABORATORY CONTINUING EDUCATION

Clinical and laboratory continuing education must include training in critical care issues as they relate to adult, pediatric, and neonatal patients. The education should also provide information that covers emergency care for the trauma patient as well as labor and delivery protocols. Lab tests required for invasive procedures should be readdressed, and information about the pre-hospital experience should be covered. Additionally, the transport team should participate in regular recertification programs from the American Heart Association on the topics of Basic Life Support (BLS), Advanced Cardiac Life Support (ACLS), Pediatric Advanced Life Support (PALS), and Neonatal Resuscitation Program (NRP). Certification in Advanced Trauma Life Support (ATLS) should also be documented. Nursing certifications must be up-to-date if a particular transport team member position description requires the training.

EDUCATING THE PUBLIC ABOUT ROLE OF FLIGHT TRANSPORT PROGRAMS IN THE HEALTHCARE SYSTEM

The transport team can educate the public about flight transport programs in a number of ways. They can offer presentations to civic groups throughout their community; these presentations can provide an overview about the types of trauma, critical care, and specialty transport services the program has available. Furthermore, they can sponsor health-related programs and offer them to the public on topics such as injury prevention. The team can also educate the public about their program by delivering educational presentations and demonstrations to schools, which serves the dual purposes of promoting health education to students in their local communities as well as marketing the flight transport program. The media – including newspapers, radio, and television – the Internet and printed materials such as flyers and brochures are also effective avenues for getting information to the public about flight transport programs.

PROVIDING EDUCATION TO SCHOOLS

Flight transport team members participate in educational opportunities at schools by offering presentations that may include lectures, videos, and aircraft and flight team personnel demonstrations. Presentations of this sort can offer information such as ways to prevent trauma injuries, what to do when a trauma injury occurs, guidelines for maintaining safety around firearms, how to recognize signs of drug abuse, and tips to prevent drinking and driving. In any presentation delivered in a public education setting, the information presented should be relevant to the age(s) of the audience members, and it should be constructed in a manner that the information can be easily understood by the audience. One powerful way to deliver public education messages is to incorporate information – either directly or indirectly – from patients who have previously utilized flight transport services.

CUMULATIVE STRESS AND TRAUMATIC STRESS

Cumulative stress, also known as burnout, occurs when an individual lets distress – or bad stress – build up over time. Cumulative stress may be caused by a series of events or occurrences rather than one stressful event. It can cause physical as well as psychological changes in an individual. Oftentimes, cumulative stress results in a feeling of being overwhelmed with one's life. This overwhelmed, out-of-control feeling can lead to other physical symptoms such as anxiety, nervousness, and an inability to concentrate. Severe cases of cumulative stress that are left untreated can lead to depression, substance abuse, and/or loss of interest in life. Conversely, traumatic stress is stress that occurs as a reaction to a specific traumatic event or occurrence such as the unexpected death of a patient during transport. Physical and psychological reactions to traumatic stress do not typically linger in the individual after the event has ended.

PRINCIPLES OF CRISIS INTERVENTION APPROACH

Crisis intervention approaches are often used to help deal with acute stress that is brought on by a traumatic incident. The four principles that guide this approach are immediacy, proximity, expectancy, and brevity. Immediacy refers to the idea that crisis intervention support services should be provided to flight team members who are experiencing acute stress as soon as possible after the occurrence of the traumatic incident. The principle of proximity suggests that services should be offered as close as possible to the location where the incident occurred. Expectancy is a principle characterized by the need to reassure the flight team member or members dealing with acute stress that they will be able to return to their work activities as soon as the stress is controlled. The principle of brevity suggests that support services should only be offered for the amount of time necessary to get the stressful reaction under control.

CISM SYSTEM COMPONENTS

Many Critical Incident Stress Management (CISM) programs begin with an education component prior to field deployment. This education involves informing flight transport team members about stress-inducing factors common in their line of work. The education additionally provides team members with tools to help strengthen their psychological resiliency so that they can most effectively handle stressful incidents in the field. CISM programs also generally incorporate crisis intervention components that are provided at the time of a disaster. These interventions typically involve psychological decompression sessions available immediately following the critical incident; crisis management briefings presented to large groups of people as an opportunity to disseminate consistent information about the event, answer questions, and offer tools to help team members cope with the event; and follow-up interventions such as peer counseling and group discussions provided several hours or even a couple weeks after a critical event.

FAIR WORK ENVIRONMENT

A fair work environment is one in which ethics and fair treatment are priorities. The fair work environment begins with publishing, disseminating, and posting a code of ethics by which all members of the organization are expected to comply. Managers at all levels must be trained in ethics and should demonstrate unbiased and fair treatment of employees. Management should have an open-door policy or other means for those at all levels to express their concerns or suggestions to better improve the organization. Performance reviews should have the input of those being reviewed and should be equitable, based on objective standards of performance. Criteria for performance, benefits, promotion, salary increases, and disciplinary actions should be clearly stated. Employees should be paid for overtime, allowed breaks, and encouraged to maintain a balance between life and work. Bullying and harassment or anything that results in a hostile environment must not be tolerated, and safety standards must be maintained.

Resuscitation Principles

PRIMARY ASSESSMENT OF PATIENT'S BREATHING

During the primary breathing assessment, the rate and depth of the patient's respirations should be noted. Determining whether the patient's skin appears bluish – cyanotic – is another assessment component. Identifying tracheal positioning should also be part of the assessment. The flight team should note whether the patient's breathing is labored and/or whether any injury exists that may impact breathing capacity. Using muscles other than the diaphragm or the intercostal muscles for breathing should be noted, as that can signal respiratory distress. Flaring of the nostrils can be another indication of respiratory distress, and should be noted if present. The primary breathing assessment should further include an evaluation of whether breath sounds occur bilaterally, whether chest movements are symmetric, and whether abnormal sounds such as crackles or rales are present. Finally, the assessment should incorporate palpation of crepitus, which are crackling or popping sounds that occur under the patient's skin or joints.

SECONDARY ASSESSMENT OF PATIENTS

The secondary assessment is a head to toe evaluation of a patient. Inspection, palpation, and auscultation provide information about the patient during the evaluation. First, the secondary assessment should include an evaluation of the overall appearance of the patient; this appearance evaluation should include an assessment of the patient in relation to his/her environment. The flight team should observe whether the patient is cognizant of his/her surroundings and how he/she interacts with them. In addition to assessing the patient's general appearance and understanding of his/her environment, the flight team should evaluate the patient's skin; head and neck; eyes, ears, and nose; mouth and throat; thorax, lungs, and cardiovascular functioning; abdomen; genitourinary system; and arms, legs, and back. Skin color and temperature, sensory functioning, cavity drainage, lacerations, injuries, breath and heart sounds, pelvic tenderness, bleeding, and pulses are examples of things the flight team should examine during the secondary assessment.

AVPU METHOD FOR EVALUATING CONSCIOUSNESS LEVEL

The AVPU assessment is a quick assessment done to determine the patient's level of consciousness. This may be one of the first assessments done when initially attending a patient.

AVPU (Alert, Voice, Pain, Unresponsive)

A	Alert and awake, aware of person, place, time, and condition. Follows commands. Pediatric: active and responds to external stimuli and caregiver.	Yes	No
V	Responds to verbal stimuli, but eyes do not open spontaneously. Pediatric: Responds only when caregiver calls name.	Yes	No
P	Responds to painful stimuli, such as pinching the skin/earlobe, but not verbal. Pediatric: Responds only to painful stimuli, such as pinching nailbed.	Yes	No
U	Unresponsive, does to respond to painful or verbal stimuli. Pediatric: Unresponsive.	Yes	No

AMPLE MNEMONIC DEVICE FOR GATHERING PATIENT HISTORY

AMPLE is a mnemonic device that can assist flight team members when they attempt to collect information related to a patient's injury or medical condition. The "A" refers to the need to collect information about whether the patient has any Allergies or whether he/she has a history of – or currently uses – Alcohol or other substances. The "M" refers to the need to gather information about any Medications the patient may be taking; collecting information about immunizations is especially essential when treating a pediatric patient. The "P" denotes the patient's Past medical history, which should include information about any serious illnesses or injuries in his/her past. The "L" refers to the need to determine the patient's Last meal. Finally, the "E" denotes Events that led up to the emergency; such events would include any occurrences that took place prior to the transport team's arrival.

AREAS OF ASSESSMENT ON CHEST X-RAYS

After ensuring that the film being viewed belongs to the patient in question, a systematic approach should be used to interpret a chest x-ray. Soft tissues should be assessed for the presence of foreign bodies and/or air, and bones should be examined for fractures. The width of the mediastinum, a group of chest structures between the lungs, should be evaluated, and masses on the structures should be documented. The shape and width of the patient's heart should be assessed from the chest x-ray, and any masses visible on the trachea or hilum should be identified as well. The size of the pulmonary arteries should be evaluated, and enlargement should be documented. Assessment of a chest x-ray should also include an examination for conditions such as pleural effusion and thickening or calcification of the pleura. Lung tissue should be examined as well to determine the presence of any abnormal shadowing.

SPINAL X-RAYS
NORMAL AND ABNORMAL RESULTS

On a normal spinal x-ray, the bones of the spine – the vertebrae – do not have any abnormalities in terms of size, shape, or appearance. Additionally, a normal spinal x-ray contains no indications of fractures or dislocations. Upon assessment of the soft tissues surrounding the vertebrae, no foreign objects or air are detected in a normal spinal x-ray. Finally, the curvature of the spine appears to be typical. In contrast, abnormal results of a spinal x-ray may reveal the presence of fractures or dislocations as well as the presence of foreign bodies or air in the soft tissues. Conditions that cause abnormal curvature of the spine, such as scoliosis, can generally be seen on a spinal x-ray. Decreased bone density may be detected as well, indicating the presence of a condition such as arthritis or osteoporosis. When a spinal x-ray reveals narrow space between vertebrae, disc disease may be indicated.

TYPES

Four common types of spinal x-rays provide various pictures of the 33 bones – vertebrae – that comprise a patient's spinal column. Cervical spine x-rays provide images of the seven cervical bones, which are located in a patient's neck. The lumbosacral spine x-ray offers a picture of the five bones in a patient's lower back, known as the lumbar vertebrae, as well as the five bones that are fused together at the sacrum, the triangular bone at the base of the spine. While the view of the five bones fused at the sacrum is limited on a lumbosacral spine x-ray, the sacrum/coccyx spine x-ray provides a more detailed view of those five bones. Additionally, the sacrum/coccyx spine x-ray produces an image of the four fused bones of the coccyx, or tailbone. A thoracic spine x-ray produces pictures of the 12 bones of the chest, the thoracic bones.

NORMAL RANGES FOR MEASUREMENTS PROVIDED THROUGH A CBC

While measurements provided through a complete blood count (CBC) can vary between sexes and between laboratories, general guidelines do exist regarding normal ranges for certain measurements. The normal range for a white blood cell (WBC) count, which is measured in cells per cubic millimeter (cmm) of blood, is 4,300 to 10,000 cells per cmm. Measured in millions per cmm of blood, the normal range for a red blood cell (RBC) count is 4.2 to 6.1 million cells per cmm. Hemoglobin, which is measured in grams per deciliter (g/dL) of blood, normally ranges from 12 to

16 g/dL for females and from 13 to 18 g/dL for males. Hematocrit is measured as a percentage (%) and normally ranges from 39% to 49% for males and from 35% to 45% for females. Platelets generally range from 150,000 to 400,000 platelets per cmm of blood.

I-STAT CHEM 8+

There are many point of care testing devices on the market today. The most used device for comprehensive blood analysis is the i-STAT CHEM 8+, which includes Na, K, Cl, Ionized Ca, CO_2, anion gap, glucose, creatinine, urea nitrogen, hemoglobin and hematocrit.

H&H	Decrease may indicate anemia, bleeding, certain cancers, chronic kidney disease
BUN/Creatinine	Kidney function: Increases with kidney disease.
Carbon dioxide (CO_2)	Measures bicarbonate. Increase may indicate breathing disorder, excessive vomiting. Decrease may indicate metabolic, lactic, or keto- acidosis, aspirin overdose, methanol poisoning.
Anion Gap	High: Toxins, Acidosis, Renal Failure
Glucose	Blood sugar level. Increase can indicate DKA while decrease can indicate insulin reaction.
Serum chloride	Increase may indicate metabolic acidosis, respiratory alkalosis, bromide poisoning. Decrease may indication burns, Addison's disease, respiratory acidosis, metabolic alkalosis, CHF dehydration.
Serum potassium	Increase may indicate tissue injury, kidney failure, respiratory/metabolic acidosis. Decrease may indicate diarrhea/vomiting, diet issues, overuse of diuretics.
Serum sodium	High: excess sweating, diarrhea, burns, or use of diuretics. Low: dehydration, vomiting, diarrhea.

CAUSES OF BILIRUBIN, BLOOD, GLUCOSE, AND PROTEIN IN URINE

Bilirubin is typically excreted into bile by the liver; consequently, liver disease can be indicated when bilirubin is present in a patient's urine. Bilirubin in urine may also indicate that a patient's gall bladder is not functioning properly. Blood in a patient's urine can be particularly serious, as it can indicate a number of possible medical complications. When a patient's urinalysis reveals blood, the blood can be an indicator of an infection or kidney stones, and it can also be an indicator of trauma or bleeding from organs such as the bladder. The presence of glucose in a patient's urine may indicate diabetes; however, it is important to note that a small number of patients do show glucose upon urinalysis without actually having diabetes. A urinalysis that indicates the presence of protein may be a sign of kidney damage or an infection.

GENERAL INDICATIONS FOR PATIENT TRANSPORT

While no universally-accepted guidelines govern indications for patient transport, general indications do exist. The decision about whether a patient should be transported from one facility to another or from a field site to a healthcare facility generally depends on the extent of the patient's injuries or illness. Time and distance also play roles in making the determination whether to transport a patient. Oftentimes, the terrain and the weather dictate whether transport services can be provided to a patient. If the patient is already at a healthcare facility, the decision to move him/her to a different facility is typically based on whether the patient can receive necessary procedures and expert care at the referring facility. Additionally, sometimes patient transport can be indicated if the patient's family requests such a transfer.

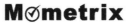

ACS Indications for Transporting Patients with Chest Injuries

According to the American College of Surgeons (ACS), patients with chest injuries may be acceptable transport candidates depending on the severity of the injury or injuries they have sustained. Patients who have a widened mediastinum may require transport; the mediastinum is a group of chest structures between the lungs that are enveloped by loose connective tissue. Transport is also indicated when a patient presents with a pulmonary contusion – a bruised lung – as the injury can potentially become quite serious and, in some patients, can lead to death. Additionally, the ACS recommends transport for patients whose chest injuries necessitate ventilation management for a prolonged period of time.

Transferring Patients Who Are Not Stabilized

According to the Consolidated Omnibus Budget Reconciliation Act (COBRA), the benefits of transferring a patient who is not stabilized need to outweigh the potential risks he/she may incur from a transfer; this must be certified in writing by the transferring physician. Second, prior to transfer, the transferring hospital should treat the patient to the best of its ability in order to decrease potential risks to the patient during transfer. Third, the receiving facility must agree to have the patient transferred to their facility; in agreeing to do so, the receiving facility is acknowledging that it has space and personnel to care for the patient. Fourth, the transferring facility must provide the receiving hospital with all available medical records associated with the patient being transferred. Finally, qualified personnel and transport equipment must be available to facilitate the patient transfer.

Patient Assessment and Management During Transport

While a patient's injuries generally dictate his/her assessment and management, certain principles can be applied to all situations. During transport, flight team members should always maintain a position that allows for efficient management of the patient's airway, breathing, and circulation. Airway equipment and all lines – intravenous (IV), central, and intraosseous – should be easy to access and in proper working order. Tubes and drainage systems should also be in proper working order; additionally, they should be secured in a manner that helps prevent displacement. If any uncertainty exists about whether a cervical spine injury is present, the cervical spine should be immobilized. Combative patients should be restrained appropriately. Medical monitors aboard the aircraft should be located in positions where the flight team members can easily view them. Finally, wounds and injured limbs should be left exposed during transport in order for the flight team to continually evaluate such injuries.

PHI

The Prehospital Index (PHI) is a measurement tool used to help triage patients in the field who have experienced some level of trauma. The PHI looks at the patient's systolic blood pressure, pulse and respiratory rates, level of consciousness, and chest and/or abdominal wounds to help determine the level of care the patient requires. For each of the aforementioned parameters of the PHI, a point score is assigned. The PHI is the total of the combined point scores for systolic blood pressure, pulse rate, respirations, consciousness, and penetrating wounds; the PHI can range from zero points to 24 points. If a patient's PHI is three points or less, it indicates minor trauma; major trauma is indicated by a PHI greater than three points.

CRAMS Scale

The CRAMS Scale examines five patient parameters to determine whether the patient needs to be transported to a trauma center. The five parameters of the CRAMS Scale are: 1) circulation; 2) respiratory rate; 3) abdominal examination; 4) motor skills; and 5) speech skills. Each parameter is scored on a scale from zero to two; patients are given scores of "two" when the parameter being examined is normal. A patient's total CRAMS Scale score – the combined score from each individual parameter score – can range from zero to 10, with 10 indicating patients exhibiting minor trauma symptoms and zero indicating patients who have sustained major trauma. Patients whose CRAMS Scale score is eight or less should be transported to a trauma facility.

PQRST METHOD TO EVALUATE PAIN LEVEL

The PQRST method is used to obtain a patient's pain history. The P represents "provoking factors." The Q represents the pain "quality." The R represents "region and radiation" of the pain. The S represents the pain "severity." The T represents "time" in relation to the pain. Flight team members should assess provoking factors in terms of the pain. The patient should identify whether specific movements or activities make the pain less or more severe. Asking the patient to describe the qualities and characteristics of the pain may provide information about where the pain originates. The patient should be asked to identify the area(s) on his/her body where the pain radiates. Using a scale of one to 10 – with 10 being most severe – the patient should be asked to categorize his/her level of pain. Finally, the patient should identify what time the pain began and how long the pain has existed.

MANAGING PAIN DURING TRANSPORT

Several techniques can be employed to help patients manage pain during transport. One effective pain management tool is distraction; providing the patient with an opportunity to think of something other than the pain can help alleviate it to an extent. With pediatric patients, security objects such as blankets and stuffed animals can often distract them and take their thoughts off the pain. Simply engaging the patient in everyday conversation can also provide a distraction for him/her, which might help the patient manage the pain. Maintaining the patient in a comfortable position as well as regulating his/her body temperature to a comfortable level are often effective pain management strategies. When clinical processes need to be performed during transport, the patient's pain can often be managed by having such processes explained to him/her. If appropriate and feasible, having a family member accompany the patient can also help the patient deal with his/her pain.

LOWERING RISK OF HEAT LOSS PRIOR TO TRANSPORT

Prior to transport, several measures should be initiated to reduce a patient's risk of heat loss, which can quickly lead to the development of hypothermia. First, the patient should be covered with a blanket to provide insulation. If examinations need to be performed in the field prior to transport, the amount of skin exposure a patient is subjected to needs to be limited. Additionally, the flight team should ensure that the patient is shielded from wind created by the rotor blades on the aircraft. During transport, it is important that the flight team keeps the patient away from metal, as metal has the ability to draw heat away from the patient's body. Finally, oxygen and fluids administered intravenously may be given to the patient to help reduce heat loss.

PRIMARY ASSESSMENT OF AIRWAY

When assessing a patient's airway, a determination should be made as to whether the airway is patent – characterized by the patient being awake and alert and having the ability to speak; able to be maintained; or not able to be maintained. The patient's level of consciousness should also be evaluated when assessing his/her airway, as the consciousness level can provide an indication of how effectively the airway is functioning. The appearance of the patient's skin should be determined during the airway assessment as well; the presence of ashen, gray or bluish, pale, or blotchy skin should be noted. During the airway assessment, a determination should be made as to the most effective way to position the patient in order to maintain his/her airway. Additionally, sounds of obstruction in the airway should be identified and noted.

LMA USE IN TRANSPORT SETTING

ADVANTAGES

One of the greatest advantages of using a laryngeal mask airway (LMA) as an airway management tool in a transport setting is that it does not require a great deal of skill or training to effectively use the device. Additionally, LMAs do not require that the patient's head and neck be moved around much, and they can be inserted with the flight team member positioned either in front of or behind the patient. These advantages make LMAs a particularly good choice in transport settings where the patient may be entrapped and/or difficult to reach, such as motor vehicle accidents. Unlike many other airway management tools, LMAs are available in sizes appropriate for pediatric patients, which is another advantage they offer. Furthermore, LMAs may not irritate patients' throats as much as other methods of intubation can, which is a particularly attractive benefit to patients.

CONTRAINDICATIONS

In order to use a laryngeal mask airway (LMA), the patient must be either unconscious or heavily sedated; consequently, patients who are alert and/or aware are not good candidates for LMAs. Additionally, an LMA does not offer any protection against aspiration of stomach contents; therefore, using an LMA is not advisable with patients who may have full stomachs, as the contents could be sucked into the lungs and cause further medical complications. It is also not advisable to utilize an LMA with patients who exhibit signs of poor pulmonary compliance, with patients who present with problems with their larynx, or with patients who have any kind of abnormalities related to their pharynx.

SECURING AN AIRWAY VIA ENDOTRACHEAL INTUBATION

Apnea – brief pauses in a patient's breathing pattern – and/or respiratory insufficiency – whereby oxygen supply and carbon dioxide removal are inadequate – can be indications for securing an airway via endotracheal intubation. If a patient's upper airway is obstructed, endotracheal intubation is likely necessary as well. Patients with an altered level of consciousness are often intubated with an endotracheal tube in an attempt to protect their airway from potential damage or injury; additionally, patients with other conditions that could potentially compromise their airways are likely to have an endotracheal tube placed as well. Endotracheal intubation is also indicated in patients experiencing increased intracranial pressure, those with hemodynamic instability, and patients presenting with signs of shock.

ORAL INTUBATION

The first step in oral intubation is to position the patient. Those not categorized as trauma patients should have their neck flexed forward with their head extended backward while trauma patients should be in a position of in-line traction. After preoxygenating the patient, the flight team member performing the intubation should open the patient's mouth with one hand while holding a laryngoscope in the other. The laryngoscope blade should be inserted in the right side of the patient's mouth, his/her tongue should be moved to the left, and the blade should be moved toward landmarks. Cricoid pressure should be applied once the epiglottis and vocal cords are displayed. Using the largest tube possible, the tube should pass from the right corner of the patient's mouth through his/her vocal cords. Once the stylet has been removed, the tube cuff can be inflated. After confirming proper positioning, the tube should be secured.

NASAL INTUBATION

The first steps in nasal intubation are to evaluate nasal patency and anesthetize the patient's nasal passages. Trauma patients should be maintained in a position of in-line traction while those not categorized as trauma patients can either sit upright or lie down with their neck flexed slightly forward and their head extended slightly backward. Oxygen should be supplied to the patient, and the intubation tube should be lubricated. As the flight team member performing the intubation advances the tube into the nasal septum, he/she should listen to the patient's breath sounds coming through the other end of the tube. On inspiration, the tube should be passed quickly into the patient's trachea. Another flight team member assisting with the procedure should apply cricoid pressure to align the glottic opening. After confirming proper positioning, the tube should be secured.

POSSIBLE COMPLICATIONS FROM NASAL ENDOTRACHEAL TUBE

Paranasal sinusitis, a condition characterized by one or more of the paranasal sinuses becoming infected, can result if the nasal endotracheal tube impedes normal drainage. Sepsis is another illness that can occur while a nasal endotracheal tube is in place. Sepsis is characterized by a bacterial infection in the bloodstream and often occurs in patients with already compromised immune systems or existing medical conditions. The infection can quickly turn fatal without proper treatment. Bacteremia is a condition characterized by bacteria in the bloodstream. Unlike sepsis, bacteremia is generally not serious and often does not require treatment. Another complication that can occur when a nasal endotracheal tube is in place is turbinate damage; turbinates are bony structures on each side of the nose that augment its ability to filter air. Nasal necrosis – death of tissue in the nasal passages – can also occur while a nasal endotracheal tube is in place.

ADVANTAGES OF PERFORMING NASAL INTUBATION VS. ORAL INTUBATION

While oral intubation is the most common method of managing a patient's airway, nasal intubation is a fairly simple, well-tolerated procedure that offers advantages over oral intubation. Nasal tubes are easier to secure than oral tubes; consequently, the chance of dislodging an oral tube is greater than the chance of dislodging a nasal one. For patients with an injured neck or jaw, a nasal tube is easier to insert than an oral one. Additionally, nasal intubation is more comfortable for patients who are awake during the procedure; it is also more comfortable when a patient awakens with a nasal tube in place as opposed to an oral tube. Patients with nasal tubes are not able to bite the tube, which can cause added medical complications. Furthermore, nasal intubation allows simultaneous surgery within the oral cavity, if necessary; such surgery is more complicated to perform around an oral tube.

CONFIRMING PROPER TUBE PLACEMENT WITH ORAL AND NASAL INTUBATION

Direct observation of the ETT passing through the vocal cords on video laryngoscope is the best confirmation of correct placement. However, there are other techniques that can be assessed together to reliably confirm tube placement. Upon auscultation over the patient's axilla – the armpit – and chest, hearing bilateral breath sounds is suggestive that an oral tube is in the correct location. Additionally, upon auscultation over the patient's epigastrium, which is located along his/her abdominal wall above the belly button, the absence of any gurgling sounds indicates that the oral tube was placed properly. Symmetric movements of the patient's chest wall will also verify placement. In pediatric patients, an appropriate pulse rate, which can be tracked on a cardiac monitor, can imply proper oral tube positioning; improved coloring in pediatric patients is another effective indicator of proper placement. Upon auscultation over the patient's chest, bilateral breath sounds will confirm proper tube placement from a nasal intubation. Symmetric movements of the patient's chest wall will also verify appropriate placement. Accurate nasal tube placement can also be verified by ensuring that the patient cannot speak. All these used in conjunction with general patient assessment and hemodynamic monitoring can help to confirm placement when video laryngoscopy isn't possible.

RSI

PROCEDURE

Once the need for rapid sequence intubation (RSI) has been established, a brief neurological assessment should be performed on the patient. Upon completion of the neurological exam, the patient should be preoxygenated for two to four minutes with 100 percent oxygen. During the preoxygenation process, positive pressure ventilation should be avoided. After administering oxygen to the patient, premedications and induction agents should be administered. Cricoid pressure should be applied once the patient loses consciousness, which is indicated by the lack of a lash reflex. A neuromuscular blocking agent should be administered next, and then the patient should be intubated when apnea is detected. At this point, the cuff should be inflated and the patient should receive 100 percent oxygen. After confirming proper placement of the endotracheal tube, cricoid pressure should be released, and the tube should be secured.

INDICATIONS

Rapid sequence intubation (RSI) is performed on patients who need a secure airway in a rapid manner; it involves simultaneous anesthesia and intubation. RSI is indicated in patients with head injuries, as effective airway management is crucial in such situations. Patients who overdose on drugs often require RSI to prevent their airways from becoming compromised as a result of the overdose. Patients presenting with status epilepticus – a condition characterized by the occurrence of a prolonged seizure or two or more seizures that occur in close succession to one another – generally require RSI, as the condition can lead to brain damage or death quite quickly; consequently, it is essential that patients with status epilepticus have a secure airway to maximize their chances for survival. Other indications for RSI include patients who are agitated or combative and those who cannot open their mouths completely, which is a condition referred to as trismus. Two intravenous lines should be in place before RSI and the patient preoxygenated for 3 minutes or more. Sellick's maneuver (pressure applied externally with thumb and index finger to the cricoid) is used to close off the esophagus and prevent aspiration. An induction agent is followed by a muscle relaxant. Sixty seconds after the muscle relaxant, an endotracheal tube is inserted with a laryngoscopy, cuff inflated, secured, and placement verified by capnometer.

DOSE, ONSET, AND DURATION OF NEUROMUSCULAR BLOCKING AGENTS

The dose for cisatracurium is 0.05 to 0.2 milligrams per kilogram (mg/kg). The dose for pancuronium is 0.07 to 0.1 mg/kg. The dose for rocuronium is 0.3 to 1.2 mg/kg. The dose for vecuronium is 0.05 to 0.1 milligrams per kilogram (mg/kg). While the onset time for rocuronium is one to two minutes, the other three most common neuromuscular blocking agents each have an onset time of three to five minutes. With a duration of 60 to 90 minutes, pancuronium is considered a prolonged blockade. In contrast, the other three agents each last a considerably shorter period of 20 to 35 minutes.

INDUCTION AGENTS

Etomidate (pregnancy Category C) is commonly used for induction for rapid sequence intubation (RSI) but has no analgesic properties. Dosage is 0.3 mg/kg IV over 30-60 seconds. Onset of action is 15 to 45 seconds and duration is 3 to 12 minutes. Etomidate has few cardiovascular effects, so it is often preferred for cardiac or hypotensive patients. Adverse effects include transient apnea, depression of cortisol level for up to 8 hours, and local pain at injection site. Etomidate is contraindicated for patients <10 and nursing mothers. Geriatric patients may require lower dosages.

Ketamine (pregnancy Category B) may be used for induction for RSI for patients who are hypotensive or having bronchospasms and for babies 3-12 months, children, pregnant women, and adults. Dosage is 1 to 2 mg/Kg IV to a maximum single dose of 500 mg for adults. Onset of action is less than 30 seconds, and duration is only 5 to 15 minutes although full recovery may take hours. Emergence reactions can include hallucinations, delirium, and disturbing dreams. Contraindications include significant hypertension and drug sensitivity.

Midazolam (pregnancy Category D) is a benzodiazepine for rapid sequence intubation (RSI). Dosage is 0.1 to 0.3 mg/kg per IV push over 2 minutes. Onset of action is 30 to 60 seconds, and duration is 15 to 30 minutes. Midazolam does not have analgesic properties but does have anticonvulsive properties, so it is indicated for status epilepticus. Adverse effects include hypotension, so midazolam is usually contraindicated in the presence of shock or hypovolemia. Other adverse effects include respiratory and cardiac arrest.

Propofol (pregnancy Category B) is the most commonly used anesthetic agent for children and adults and can be used as an induction agent for RSI. Propofol reduces airway resistance and is appropriate for patients with bronchospasm. It also has neuro-inhibitory effects, so it can reduce ICP in patients with intracranial pathology. Dosage is 1.5 to 3 mg/kg IV with onset of action within 15 to 45 seconds and duration 5 to 10 minutes. Adverse effects include cardiac and respiratory depression and hypotension. Contraindicated in patients with allergies to eggs or soybeans.

VIDEO LARYNGOSCOPE TECHNOLOGY

The video laryngoscope is a battery-powered laryngoscope with a light source and built in camera, usually near the distal end of the blade to facilitate intubation. It is especially helpful with a difficult airway, allowing indirect viewing of the larynx. Various blades are available, including hyper-angulated, channeled (to guide the endotracheal tube), and the standard Macintosh blade. The blade is inserted into the mouth as with a standard laryngoscope and settled into the vallecula. The epiglottis and vocal chords are viewed through the monitor, which is mounted on the handle. However, the field of vision is closer with the camera than the eye, so the CFRN should never depend just on the monitor when inserting the ETT. An alternative method of doing a video laryngoscope is to thread an ETT over a fiberoptic scope for intranasal insertion. Once the scope is in the trachea, the ETT is advanced and the scope withdrawn.

NEEDLE CRICOTHYROTOMY

A needle cricothyrotomy is typically performed as a last resort when all other attempts to secure an airway have failed. It is often done as an emergency procedure to manage an airway obstruction until a tracheostomy can be performed. Skin should be prepped with an antiseptic solution and if the situation doesn't permit it, local anesthetic like 1% lidocaine can be given with a 27 g needle. During procedure monitor vitals and respirations. Universal precautions and sterile technique should be used. The patient's head should be placed in a stable, neutral position. With the thumb and middle finger of non-dominant hand, hold tension of skin and trachea in place while using the index finger to feel the thyroid membrane. Using a 10 cc syringe that is half filled with saline and attached to an over the needle IV catheter held in dominant hand, insert the needle midline in the neck at the lowest margin of the thyroid membrane and angle it toward the feet at about a 45 degree angle. While puncturing the skin and underlying tissue, pull back on the syringe while advancing the catheter and needle until air bubbles can be seen. Advance catheter off the needle and rest its hub on the skin (this part of the skill is similar to IV catheter advancement after getting flashback). To confirm placement you can reattach the syringe to the catheter and aspirate, expecting air return. Have the catheter held firmly in place while high pressure oxygen tubing is connected and the catheter is secured in place with sutures.

RAPID FOUR-STEP CRICOTHYROTOMY TECHNIQUE

The Rapid Four-Step Cricothyrotomy Technique involves palpation, incision, traction, and intubation. First, the patient's cricoid membrane is palpated while his/her trachea is palpated and stabilized. Next, a horizontal incision is made in the patient's cricothyroid membrane using a scalpel held at a 60-degree angle; the incision should be approximately two and a half centimeters (cm) in length. The scalpel should be left in place once the incision has been made. Third, a tracheal hook is placed against the blade of the scalpel and guided down the trachea. In an inferior direction, the tracheal hook's tip should be rotated 90 degrees, and traction should be applied to the cricoid cartilage. At this point, the examiner places his/her hand on the patient's sternum to maintain tracheal traction while the scalpel is removed. Finally, the examiner intubates the patient, and the tracheal hook is removed once correct placement of the tube is confirmed.

ESTABLISHING A SURGICAL AIRWAY

The establishment of a surgical airway may be indicated in a patient whose airway is inaccessible by alternate means. Patients who suffer trauma around their airway may be difficult to intubate using orotracheal or nasotracheal methods, as trauma can cause anatomy deformities and/or extensive bleeding that can inhibit visualization of the airway. Establishing a surgical airway may also be necessary in patients whose upper airways are entirely obstructed. Foreign objects, mass lesions, and edema – swelling of an organ or tissue as a result of lymph fluid build-up – can all lead to upper airway obstruction. Situations where the establishment of a surgical airway may be counter-indicated include those involving patients younger than 10 years old, those involving patients where the flight team is not able to identify landmarks for puncture purposes, and those involving patients who have either a puncture site infection or a primary injury to their larynx.

TRACHEOSTOMY
POSSIBLE COMPLICATIONS

Respiratory distress is a common complication of a tracheostomy. Mucus plugs or other forms of tracheostomy (trach) tube obstruction are often the cause of respiratory distress; such obstructions can generally be eliminated through suctioning the trach tube. Given that a tracheostomy opening is made by a surgical incision, the chance of developing an infection around the incision site exists. Pneumothorax, a condition which occurs when air or gas collects outside the patient's lungs, can also be a post-operative complication of a tracheostomy. Signs of the condition may include shortness of breath, cyanosis, and an increased heart rate. Pneumomediastinum, a condition that occurs when air collects in the mediastinum, a group of chest structures between the lungs, is another potential tracheostomy complication. Although rare, bleeding can occur as a complication during the actual procedure.

SUCTIONING

With clean and/or gloved hands, the individual performing the tracheostomy suctioning should pick up the catheter at the end closest to the suction machine; the end that will be placed in the trach tube should not be handled. The catheter should then be attached to the tube on the suction machine, and the machine should be started. Identify how far the catheter should be inserted into the tracheostomy (trach) tube; it should generally be inserted to a point equivalent to the length of the tube plus an additional quarter inch. After identifying the stopping point, the catheter should be advanced into the trach tube. At this point, suction is applied when the individual performing the suctioning places his/her thumb over the catheter's hole while removing it from the trach tube. As the catheter is pulled out, the individual performing the suctioning should roll the tube between his/her thumb and forefinger.

ADVANTAGES OF USING A MECHANICAL VENTILATOR

One of the main advantages of using a mechanical ventilator is the consistency it offers in various areas. Mechanical ventilators provide consistent volumes of gas inhaled and exhaled during each cycle of respiration, known as tidal volumes. Furthermore, ventilation rates – or breathing rates – can be maintained in a consistent manner using a mechanical ventilator. Another area in which mechanical ventilators offer consistency is the concentration of oxygen they deliver to the patient. Additionally, unlike manual ventilation, which requires healthcare professionals to use their hands during the process of ventilating a patient, mechanical ventilators allow them to utilize their hands for other clinical tasks.

CONTINUOUS WAVEFORM CAPNOGRAPHY FOR INTUBATED PATIENTS

Capnography measures exhaled carbon dioxide and may include a capnometer, which provides a numeric CO_2 measure, or a capnogram, which provides a visual waveform. End tidal CO_2 ($ETCO_2$ or $PETCO_2$) is the partial pressure of CO_2 at the end of expiration. The normal $ETCO_2$ is 35 to 45 mmHg, and waveforms should be consistent. Capnography is more sensitive than pulse oximetry, which changes more slowly in the presence of apnea. Capnography is used initially to confirm correct placement of an ETT. Once intubated, patients should be monitored with continuous waveform capnography. Decreased perfusion from decreased cardiac output or pulmonary blood flow results in decreased CO_2 level and hypoventilation in increased CO_2. If a notch occurs in the waveform, this can indicate the patient is arousing from sedation or beginning to breathe independently. Capnography should be monitored during and after position change and transfers to ensure that the ETT is not dislodged.

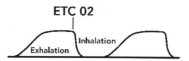

INITIAL MECHANICAL VENTILATION SETTINGS

Ventilation settings will vary according to the size and condition of the patient, but typical initial ventilation settings include:

- Tidal volume: The maximum is 10 mL/kg of ideal body weight (IBW) if patient has no lung disease but must be kept under 10 mL/Kg IBW if lung disease is present.
- Pressure: Initially 20 to 25 cm H_2O and then adjusted to maintain the tidal volume.
- Respiration rate: Initially 12-16 bpm although patients with ALI/ARDS need a higher setting of 18-22 bpm.
- FiO2: Initially 100% and the adjusted to a goal of oxygen saturation ≥88% or PaO2 >55 mmHg.
- PEEP: Initially 5 cm H_2O and increased by 2 to 3 cm every 30 to 60 minutes.
- Inspiratory time: Initially 0.8 to 1 second.
- I:E ratio: Initially 1:2 and then adjusted to 1:3 or 1:4 or other settings appropriate for patient.

Ventilation should generally be adjusted to maintain the patient's normal or baseline PCO_2. If oxygenation is inadequate, the FiO_2 and/or PEEP should be increased. If ventilation needs to be increased because of falling CO_2, the respiration rate or tidal volume should be increased.

SIMV MODE OF MECHANICAL VENTILATION

The synchronized intermittent mandatory ventilation (SIMV) model of mechanical ventilation is a combination mode in which the ventilator delivers mandatory breaths synchronized with the patient's effort of breathing but allows spontaneous breaths between the mandatory breaths. In the SIMV phase, if a patient triggers a breath at all, the ventilator delivers a preset tidal volume to ensure adequate ventilation. In the mandatory part of the SIMV phase, if the patient does not trigger a breath within the first 90% of the SIMV phase, a mandatory breath is automatically delivered. If the patient breathes spontaneously, the ventilator is not triggered although the ventilator can be set to provide some tidal volume in support of spontaneous breaths that are not adequate. The SIMV mode is often used when weaning a patient from mechanical ventilation.

MODES OF VENTILATION

Modes of ventilation include:

- Assist control: The patient receives a preset tidal volume during each inspiration, whether the breath is triggered by the individual or by the ventilator. The mandatory breath occurs at a preset duration of time after the previous inspiration if the patient does not trigger a spontaneous breath. Assist control is the most commonly utilized mode of ventilation.
- Continuous mandatory ventilation: The patient receives a preset tidal volume at a preset rate, so the patient cannot trigger ventilation with spontaneous breaths. This mode is commonly used for patient who are paralyzed and during surgery when patients have received muscle relaxants.
- Pressure support ventilation: The ventilator delivers a preset level of inspiratory pressure in support of a patient's inspiratory effort. The frequency, duration, and tidal volume are determined by the patient, so the machine should be set with backup settings in the event of apnea if possible.

CHEST COMPRESSION IN CPR

Excellent chest compressions are the cornerstone of good CPR. Allow chest recoil, minimize interruptions, and maintain depth and rate.

	Adult	**Child**	**Infant**
Age	Past puberty	1 y/o - puberty	Under 1
Compressions to Ventilations	30:2	15:2	15:2
Chest Compression rate	At least 100/minute	At least 100/minute	At least 100/minute
Chest Compression Land Marking Method	two hands center of the chest, even with nipples	one hand center of the chest even with nipples	2 or 3 fingers, just below the nipple line at the center of the chest
Chest Compression Depth	At least 2" compression (hands overlapping)	about 2" compression or 1/3 the AP diameter (only heel of one hand)	about 1 ½" compression or 1/3 the AP diameter (2 fingers)

CARDIOVERSION AND DEFIBRILLATION

Cardioversion delivers a low energy shock that is synchronized to the QRS. Defibrillation (also called unsynchronized cardioversion) gives a high energy non-synchronized shock anywhere in the cardiac cycle. While both procedures attempt to restore the natural rhythm of the heart, cardioversion is performed on individuals who are not experiencing cardiac arrest, and defibrillation is generally performed as an emergency procedure on patients who are having a heart attack. Both procedures employ electric shock as a method for restarting the heart's rhythm, but cardioversion uses much lower levels of electricity than defibrillation uses. Most cardioversions are conducted to treat atrial flutter, which is a series of stable, regular flutter waves typically ranging from 240 to 400 beats per minute, or atrial fibrillation, which is a disturbance to the heart's rhythm that begins in the atria. Cardioversion is also used to treat stable ventricular tachycardia. Defibrillation tends to be a more risky procedure because the electrical shock used actually stops the heart altogether in an attempt to restore its normal beating rhythm.

STEPS IN PERFORMING DEFIBRILLATION ON PATIENTS IN CARDIAC ARREST

High quality CPR should be performed as soon as sudden cardiac arrest is recognized and continued until the defibrillator is attached by another team member and ready to use. Interruptions in CPR should be minimized. Airway should be assessed and maintained. Power on the defibrillator. Place one pad on the upper right side of the patient's chest. The area should be right and lateral of the sternum, mid clavicular line. The posterior pad should be placed slightly sub scapular, with the center of the pad about equal with the T7 vertebrae. This is known as anterior posterior (AP) placement and allows for the maximum energy to flow. If AP placement is not possible, place the pad on the left lateral side, midaxillary line, with the bottom of the pad at about the 5th intercostal space. Pads should not be placed on top of pacemakers, body jewelry, or ports. Attach leads to defibrillator pads and charge defibrillator while continuing chest compressions. Stop compression to check rhythm. If VF or pulseless VT, clear patient and then administer shock at 120-200J, according to manufacturer guidelines (for biphasic defibrillators). Unless there is a return of spontaneous circulation (ROSC), immediately resume CPR for 5 cycles. Use epinephrine 1 mg every 3-5 minutes while continuing CPR if pulseless VT or VF persists. After the 5 cycles, about two minutes, check rhythm, clear patient, defibrillate again. If no ROSC, begin CPR cycle again. Continue in this pattern considering causes and treating as able or until ROSC.

CARE OF PATIENTS WITH TRANSVENOUS PACING

Transvenous pacing may be temporary (most common) or permanent, and is done for hemodynamic instability and arrhythmias, such as BBB, AV block, and bradycardia. Transvenous pacing is often done temporarily if the patient cannot tolerate transcutaneous pacing or needs to be transferred. For transvenous pacing, a pacer is inserted transvenously through the right internal jugular or left subclavian vein into the right atrium or ventricle. (The right internal jugular is preferred for temporary pacing to save the left subclavian for a permanent pacemaker.) The electrode or electrodes of the pacing wire are inserted into an external battery-powered pacing generator. The insertion site should be covered with sterile transparent dressing. The patient must have continuous cardiac monitoring once capture is established. VT due to failure to sense or bradycardia due to failure to capture can occur with pacer wire damage or dislodgement, battery failure, or incorrect settings. The patient should be observed for signs of cardiac tamponade, hematoma, infection, and pneumothorax.

MANAGING PATIENT WITH CONFIRMED ASYSTOLE

Cycles of cardiopulmonary resuscitation (CPR) and rhythm checks – lasting two minutes per cycle – should be performed on asystole patients who are acceptable resuscitation candidates.

Epinephrine can be administered to the asystole patient every three to five minutes in an attempt to overcome whatever is preventing the patient's heart from beating. Airway should be assessed and managed. The cause of the asystole should be sought and treated accordingly, if possible. Most common reversible causes include: Hypoxia, hypothermia, hypokalemia (or hyperkalemia), acidosis, thrombosis, toxins, tamponade, tension pneumo. ACLS encourages using end-tidal carbon dioxide measurement and continuous waveform capnography to assess the effectiveness of CPR or detect return of spontaneous circulation. A low end-tidal carbon dioxide level following more than 20 minutes of CPR is the most objective reason to terminate resuscitation for a patient who presents with asystole and has no ROSC. Other determinants that influence decision to terminate resuscitation: long duration of resuscitation with no ROSC, questionable or long length between time of arrest and time of CPR, increased age, and severity of certain comorbidities.

CLINICAL DEATH AND BIOLOGICAL DEATH

Clinical death is defined as an absence of breathing and blood circulation. Clinical death takes place when a patient's heart fails to continue beating. As a general guideline, clinical death is not sufficient to determine death in a patient, as attempts can be made to restart the patient's heart. When clinical death occurs, cardiopulmonary resuscitation (CPR) and advanced cardiac life support (ACLS) measures will be implemented in an attempt to resuscitate the patient. Biological death is characterized by a lack of electrical activity in a patient's brain; as such, it is also referred to as brain death. The presumption behind the definition of biological death is that consciousness ends when the brain's electrical activity ceases; consequently, biological death occurs as a result of a permanent loss of consciousness.

LOW-FLOW SYSTEMS OF ADMINISTERING OXYGEN THERAPY

A nasal cannula and a simple face mask are two forms of low-flow oxygen delivery systems. A nasal cannula delivers oxygen to the patient through a flexible tube made of plastic that is inserted in his/her nostrils. Oxygen flows through a nasal cannula at the rate of one to six liters per minute. Oxygen concentration (FIO_2) using a nasal cannula ranges from about 24-44%. The nasal cannula is the most commonly used low-flow oxygen delivery system. A simple face mask, which covers the patient's nose and mouth, is another low-flow method of administering oxygen therapy. Oxygen can flow through a mask at the rate of five to eight liters per minute. Using a mask, FIO_2 can reach approximately 60 percent. When administering oxygen via a mask, the minimum flow rate should be five liters per minute to prevent reuptake of carbon dioxide.

Of note, oxygen regulators may have been calibrated for use at regular sea level. If this is the case, the flow rate will change with increasing altitude. So oxygen set to flow at 4 L/min at 8,000 feet will actually be flowing around 5.4 L/min.

HIGH-FLOW SYSTEMS OF ADMINISTERING OXYGEN THERAPY

A non-rebreather mask – one type of high-flow oxygen delivery system – covers the patient's nose and mouth; it also has a reservoir bag attached to it, which receives oxygen from the oxygen source. Oxygen flows through a non-rebreather mask at a rate greater than 10 liters per minute. With a tightly-fit mask and a reservoir bag that inflates properly, oxygen concentration (FIO_2) using a non-rebreather mask can reach 100 percent. As such, non-rebreather masks are appropriate for use in emergencies and with patients in respiratory failure. Air entrainment masks have both variable flow rates and variable FIO_2 levels that can range from 24 to 50 percent. This method is commonly used for patients whose lungs do not remove an adequate amount of carbon dioxide (CO_2), as it offers the ability to administer oxygen at high rates and to control the FIO_2 level, and the method does not result in CO_2 accumulation.

ASSESSING OXYGENATION STATUS

A patient's oxygenation status can be assessed using several factors. A pulse oximeter, a non-invasive tool used to measure the amount of oxygen in a patient's blood, may be utilized to monitor the patient's oxygen saturation level (SaO_2). The patient's consciousness level can also be determined to help assess oxygenation status. The tone of the patient's skin as well as the absence or presence of cyanosis – a condition characterized by a bluish skin tone – can also be examined as a means of assessing oxygenation status. Monitoring the patient's airway, breathing, and circulation in addition to his/her pulse are other important components of assessing whether he/she is adequately oxygenated. Finally, monitoring the patient's inhaled and exhaled concentrations of carbon dioxide (CO_2) through capnography provides a helpful indicator of oxygenation status.

PULSE OXIMETRY

Pulse oximetry is a non-invasive technique used to measure the amount of oxygen in a patient's blood. Inaccurate readings may be obtained from patients with inadequate blood flow to their tissue, such as patients experiencing shock or cardiac arrest. The technique may also have limited effectiveness on patients with hypothermia, patients with burns, and those with highly pigmented skin. It may be difficult to obtain exact pulse oximetry values from patients who are not able to maintain a fairly still position as well as from those who have vasoactive drugs in their bloodstream. Additionally, falsely high values typically occur in patients who smoke due to the carbon monoxide in cigarette smoke. A pulse oximeter may also provide inaccurate readings when it is utilized in bright ambient light, as the intensity of the light may lead to abnormally high values.

Always compare pulse oximetry readings to the clinical presentation of the patient.

NORMAL OXYGEN SATURATION VALUES

Oxygen saturation values in the range of greater than or equal to 95 percent are generally considered normal. However, for some patients, like those COPD, normal saturations may be 88-92%. While 97 to 99 percent saturation can be considered normal values for most patients, some patients may become extremely sick if their pulse oximetry values go above 97 percent. The best way to determine a patient's target oxygen saturation is to know their history and normal resting oxygen saturation, but this is not always possible. In the absence of this knowledge and signs of COPD, in an adult patient, as a general rule, patients with oxygen saturation levels below 90 percent are in need of ventilation; typically, ventilation with oxygen saturation at a level below 90 percent can be performed with a bag-valve-mask device. The most effective way to determine whether a patient is improving as a result of oxygen delivery is simply to compare pre- and post-pulse oximetry values.

ARTERIAL BLOOD GASES

Arterial blood gas studies evaluate the acidity, oxygen content, and amount of carbon dioxide (CO_2) in a patient's blood. The analysis is generally performed to evaluate respiratory diseases and other conditions that affect the functioning of a patient's pulmonary system. Kidney functioning can also be assessed through the acid-base component of an arterial blood gas study. Additionally, the analysis can provide information about how a patient is responding to oxygen therapy. Patients who sustain traumatic injuries, particularly injuries that likely affect their breathing such as head and neck trauma, also tend to have abnormal results on arterial blood gas studies. When drawing an ABG for point of care testing, determine the best arm to take the specimen from (if possible perform the Allen test and assess for AV grafts and other implanted devices). Using universal precautions, prepare site with solution per protocol (usually chlorhexidine). Palpate the radial artery with index and middle finger then locate the radial artery. Puncture skin with needle bevel at

48

45 degrees. The needle should fill with brightly colored red blood rapidly. After sample has been collected, remove needle and hold pressure for 3 minutes or longer until bleeding is stopped, consider longer for patients on anticoagulants. Immediately perform point of care testing on sample or place on ice. Reassess neuro status of extremity used and make sure there is no further bleeding at site of puncture.

NORMAL VALUES FOR ARTERIAL BLOOD GAS STUDIES

Arterial blood gas studies measure partial pressure of oxygen (PaO_2), partial pressure of carbon dioxide ($PaCO_2$), pH level, oxygen saturation level (SaO_2), and bicarbonate (HCO_3). Normal values for these measures are values obtained at sea level; altitudes greater than 3,000 feet will generally generate lower values. A normal PaO_2 level is 75 to 100 millimeters of mercury (mmHg). $PaCO_2$ level is considered normal when it falls within the range of 35 to 45 mmHg. A pH level of 7.35 to 7.45 is within the normal range. Oxygen saturation values in the range of 97 to 99 percent are generally considered normal. However, some patients consistently deliver pulse oximetry values between 93 and 97 percent, which can be considered normal for certain patients. An HCO_3 value of 22 to 26 milliequivalent per liter (mEq/liter) falls within the normal range.

If pH is less than 7.35, then acidemia (respiratory or metabolic acidosis) or if pH is greater than 7.45, then alkalemia (respiratory or metabolic alkalosis). If the pH is within normal range, there is much less chance that an acid base disorder is present, but in a few cases the pH can be normal, especially if the rest of the ABG is abnormal. This is called a mixed disorder. After assessing the PCO_2 and HCO_3, the initial change and compensatory change can be decided, leading to an understanding of the disease process being respiratory or metabolic in origin.

TRAUMA TRIAD

The trauma triad is a leading cause of death in trauma patients, usually resulting from tissue injury and severe bleeding:

- Hypothermia: Normal temperature 35.6-37° C. Trauma hypothermia—mild (34 to 36° C), moderate (32 to 34° C), and severe (<32° C). Can result in decreased cardiac output and myocardial ischemia, decreased response to epinephrine, hypoxia, and arrhythmias. With bleeding, clotting is impaired; with infection, reduces WBCs and increases risk of infection/sepsis. May be exacerbated by alcohol intoxication, older age, chronic disease, and administration of cool IV fluids/blood products.
- Acidosis: Occurs with pH <7.35 (normal is 7.35-7.45). May be metabolic as well as respiratory acidosis. May result in decreased cardiac output and response to epinephrine, hyperventilation, respiratory fatigue, decreased mental status, coma, and impaired coagulation. May result from poor tissue perfusion, excessive resuscitation with crystalloids.
- Coagulopathy: May be dilutional from fluid resuscitation with fluids or blood products that lack lost clotting factors. May also result from pre-existing anticoagulation (warfarin, heparin) or over-activation of coagulation system.

Medical Emergencies

INSPECTION AND AUSCULTATION OF PATIENT'S ABDOMEN

With the patient's abdomen exposed, observing and inspecting his/her abdominal area can provide information about the patient's medical condition(s). During inspection, the flight team member should make note of any skin abnormalities on the abdomen. Additionally, the team member should determine whether the abdomen looks swollen. Abdominal contours are typically best seen by standing at the patient's feet and looking up in the direction of the patient's head. If the abdomen appears distended, the flight team member should note whether the distension is symmetrical. Inspection can also offer information about whether the patient is comfortable moving and/or whether he/she is able to lie still. Auscultation should be performed before percussion and palpation. Note quality and frequency of sounds.

PERCUSSION AND PALPATION OF PATIENT'S ABDOMEN

Percussion should be performed before palpation, as patients with peritonitis will have pain even with percussion. To percuss the abdomen, the examiner should place one hand on the abdominal wall so that his/her middle finger is against the patient's skin. Using the tip of the middle finger of his/her other hand, the examiner should strike the joint two or three times of the middle finger of the hand that is on the patient. This process should be repeated in each quadrant of the abdomen. The flight team member should note whether tympanitic – drum-like – or dull sounds are heard; he/she should also note any pain felt by the patient during percussion. The examiner should then lightly palpate each quadrant of the patient's abdomen to identify areas of tenderness. Deeper palpation can be performed to identify abdominal masses and/or areas of extreme tenderness. It is most effective to watch the patient's face during palpation, as the patient's expressions tend to change when tenderness is encountered. A tympany sound may indicate a distended bowel while a dull sound may indicate a solid mass. In palpation, start with the abdominal quadrant with the least pain. Note tender areas, guarding, and rebound tenderness.

INSERTING A NASOGASTRIC TUBE

If the patient is alert, the nasogastric (NG) tube insertion procedure should be explained to him/her. Before beginning the procedure, the patient should be placed in a seated position at a 90-degree angle; this position is known as high-Fowler's position. Cover the patient's chest with protective padding. To determine how much of the NG tube should be passed, use the tube itself to measure the distance from the patient's nose to his/her earlobe as well as the distance from the earlobe to the xiphoid process. Combine the two measurements, and mark the combined distance on the tube. Apply lubricant to the first six inches of the tube, and begin to pass it through the patient's largest open nostril to the nasopharynx. As the tube is being passed, it should be aimed down and back. Continue passing the tube into the patient's stomach until the mark on the tube is reached.

CONFIRMING PROPER NASOGASTRIC TUBE PLACEMENT

A chest x-ray can confirm when a nasogastric (NG) tube has successfully been placed in a patient's stomach. However, if it is not possible to obtain a chest x-ray, an irrigation syringe can be used to aspirate the contents of the patient's stomach. If a salem sump tube is correctly positioned, if you instill 30 cc of warm water via syringe and area able to immediately suction back most of the water, the sump is most likely correctly placed. If the patient coughs, chokes, and/or develops a bluish skin tone – a condition known as cyanosis – while attempting to talk, the tube has likely passed through the larynx. Finally, improper tube placement may also be detected by placing the open end of the

50

tube in water; if the tube has passed through the larynx, the water will bubble. Placement should always be verified by radiology before instilling medications or formulas due to risk of placement in bronchial tree. On arrival to a facility, notify and document that new caregivers were made aware that the tube was only clinically confirmed, but will need x-ray confirmation before anything should be instilled. CFRNs should also be aware that during long interfacility transports, previously confirmed tubes can become dislodged and that their placement should be reconfirmed if needed.

ECCHYMOSIS

Ecchymosis occurs when bleeding into the skin or mucous membranes is present. Characterized by large, flat areas on the skin where blood has pooled under the tissue, ecchymoses tend to be greater than a centimeter in diameter. Ecchymoses can be quite dangerous and should always be evaluated. In order to appropriately treat an ecchymosis, it is important to recognize the difference between the condition and general skin redness or inflammation. To determine whether a patient has an ecchymosis or skin redness, slight pressure can be applied to the site of the discoloration. An ecchymosis will not blanch – turn pale and then return to its original color – when pressure is applied; conversely, inflammations of the skin will blanch when pressure is applied.

TRANSPORT CONSIDERATIONS FOR PATIENT WITH AN IABP

Before transporting patient, the CFRN should know the reason the patient has the IABP, the type/brand of pump (and have more than one set wires for that pump), have supplies to deal with any bleeding issues easily accessible, and consider ways to keep the femoral area immobile. Make sure IABP battery is fully charged and a backup battery is available. IABP should be placed in auto mode to compensate for altitude changes. The pressure bag for the system should be inflated and the transducer at the level of the phlebostatic axis. Settings, including timing, trigger, and balloon inflation should be known and checked frequently. Since most IABPs are triggered from ECG, assessing and replacing ECG electrode pads prior to transport is essential. Prior to transport, the CFRN should assess the level of helium in the helium tank. The CFRN should be familiar with the device, understand troubleshooting, and should trace all tubing and wiring, especially from console to patient, to check for blood or issue. Assessment should be done prior to transport to aircraft, after patient is set up on aircraft, with any major changes in patient status, and when alarms sound, at minimum. CFRNs should be familiar with alarms and be able to visualize alarms when noise prevents alarms from being heard. Low pressure or helium leak alarms may indicate the IABP console should be put on hold until issue is resolved. Most IABP manufacturers state the pump can be immobile <20 mins due to risk for embolus, balloon entrapment, and vascular damage.

12-LEAD ECG

The 12-lead electrocardiogram (ECG) actually comprises 10 electrodes and 12 sources of measurement. Each represents a particular orientation in space, as indicated below (RA = right arm; LA = left arm, LF = left foot):

- Bipolar limb leads (frontal plane):
  - Lead I: RA (-) to LA (+) (Right Left, or lateral)
  - Lead II: RA (-) to LF (+) (Superior Inferior)
  - Lead III: LA (-) to LF (+) (Superior Inferior)
- Augmented unipolar limb leads (frontal plane):
  - Lead aVR: RA (+) to [LA & LF] (-) (Rightward)
  - Lead aVL: LA (+) to [RA & LF] (-) (Leftward)
  - Lead aVF: LF (+) to [RA & LA] (-) (Inferior)
- Unipolar (+) chest leads (horizontal plane):

51

- o Leads V1, V2, V3: (Posterior Anterior)
- Leads V4, V5, V6:(Right Left, or lateral)

NORMAL 12-LEAD ECG

A normal 12-lead electrocardiogram (ECG) is characterized by normal sinus rhythm, which consists of p-waves each followed by a:

- QRS complex, p-wave rates of 60 to 100 beats per minute
- normal QRS axis with normal heights and widths on the p-waves
- normal PR interval; the PR interval is the number of seconds between the start of the p-wave and the start of the QRS complex
- normal QRS complex; ventricular depolarization generally occurs within 0.06 and 0.1 seconds
- normal QT interval; the QT interval is a solid indicator of ventricular repolarization; it begins when the QRS complex starts and ends when the T wave ends
- normal ST segment; a normal ST segment indicates that the whole ventricle has been depolarized
- normal T wave; the T and U waves represent repolarization of ventricles;
- normal U wave; the U wave is not always present on a normal ECG

CAPILLARY NAIL REFILL TEST

A capillary nail refill test is a measure of how much blood is flowing to a patient's tissues, which is known as tissue perfusion. The test can quickly identify whether a patient's vascular flow is normal. The skin and nail beds are a good indicator of systemic vascular resistance and shunting. The test is performed by applying direct pressure to a patient's nail bed until the nail bed turns from pink to white in color. The individual applying the pressure to the patient's nail bed will monitor how long it takes for the nail bed to return to pink, which indicates that blood has returned to the tissue. A patient whose capillary nail refill test is longer than two seconds may be suffering from hypothermia, shock, dehydration, and/or peripheral vascular disease.

JUGULAR VENOUS PRESSURE

Jugular venous pressure should be measured with the head of the patient's bed at a 45-degree angle. The patient's head should be turned to the right for accurate measurement. With the patient's head in the proper position, the examiner should identify the patient's jugular venous pulsations. Additionally, the examiner needs to locate the sternal angle, which can be found at the superior edge of the sternum. In centimeters, the examiner should then measure the distance between the identified pulsations and the patient's sternum. If this distance measures greater than four centimeters, neck vein distention is present; the distance is considered normal if it is four centimeters or less.

CHRONIC STABLE ANGINA

Chronic stable angina is the most common form in which ischemic heart disease expresses itself in patients, and ischemic heart disease is the number one cause of death in the United States. The condition is typically characterized by pressure or a heavy feeling in the patient's chest, and it is often brought about through activity. The chest discomfort associated with chronic stable angina frequently resolves itself with rest, and many patients who live with the condition are able to stop the activity or activities causing the discomfort prior to symptoms becoming severe. Clinical histories, physical examinations, electrocardiograms, and chest x-rays can often help in the assessment of chronic stable angina. However, many patients who experience bouts of the condition will have a normal physical examination, and electrocardiograms may only prove to be useful tools if the patient is exerting him/herself during testing.

MANAGEMENT OF CHEST PAIN

Management of the patient with chest pain begins with a thorough assessment, primary and secondary survey, and utilization of OPQRST and SAMPLE methods of history taking. The patient should be placed in semi-Fowler's position, especially if experiencing shortness of breath, and oxygen saturation monitored. Respiratory compromise may require supplemental oxygen, bag-valve mask assistance, PEEP, CPAP/Bi-PAP, manually-triggered ventilators (MTVs) or automatic transport ventilators (ATVs). Interventions may include:

- Aspirin (for suspected heart attack) (Bayer®, Heartline®, XORprin®, Empirin®): 325 mg chewable (preferred). Contraindicated with GI bleeding, stroke
- Nitroglycerine (for suspected angina): (Nitrodur®, Nitrolingual®, NitroMist®): 0.4 mg sublingually repeated every 3-5 minutes up to 3 doses. Contraindicated if patient has recently taken Viagra®, with stroke, or with excessive bleeding
- 3 or 12-lead ECG recorded/transmitted during pain episode
- Continuous ECG monitoring
- Blood work for initial serum biomarkers

All patients with chest pain should be transported and cardiac symptoms/ACS protocol followed.

QUESTIONS TO ASK PATIENTS EXPERIENCING CHEST PAIN

The following are the types of questions to ask a patient presenting with chest pain:

- Quality- Describe the pain. Does it feel like a burning sensation? Does it feel like a tightening sensation in your chest? Does it feel like your chest is being constricted or squeezed? (sharp, dull, ripping, tearing, quality similar to a previous episode of ischemia)
- Where is your pain located?
- Does the pain move around from location to location? Does it move from your chest into any other area of your body? (MI pain usually is diffuse and hard to localize)
- What was happening when the pain started? (pain that occurs with rest and gets progressively worse is very concerning)
- Rate your pain on a scale of 1-10.
- How quickly did the pain come on? (sudden onset may indicate pneumothorax, PE, aortic dissection, while MI pain usually has a gradual onset with increase in intensity)
- When the pain comes on, is it continuous or does it come and go?
- Have you found or done anything that reduces or eliminates the pain? (sitting up usually improves pericarditis)
- Have you found or done anything that makes the pain worse? (respirations will worsen pleuritic chest pain)
- What other symptoms are you experiencing? (dyspnea and syncopal symptoms often accompany MIs)

CONTRAINDICATIONS FOR USING FIBRINOLYTIC AGENTS IN PATIENTS PRESENTING WITH SIGNS OF AMI

In all patients that may receive thrombolytics the risk of bleeding must be considered. In a patient presenting with signs of acute myocardial infarction (AMI), flight personnel need to be aware that the presence of any of the following make the administration of fibrinolytic agents such as t-PA, r-tPA, and TNK riskier than in patients without any of these conditions.

Absolute contraindications for fibrinolytics for patients according to ACLS with STEMIs include: ischemic stroke in the last three months unless within the last three hours; active bleeding; suspected aortic dissection; significant head or face trauma in the last three months; previous intracranial hemorrhage; known malignant intracranial neoplasm or cerebral lesion.

Relative contraindications include: uncontrolled chronic hypertension; dementia; trauma with the last three weeks; major surgery within the last three weeks; CPR for more than ten minutes within the last three weeks; some patients with prior history of ischemic stroke longer than three months ago; actively ulcer; prior allergic reaction to a fibrinolytic or streptokinase exposure within the last five days; recent internal bleeding; high INR from anticoagulant use; pregnancy. ACLS and other organizations have a fibrinolytic checklists for STEMIs to promote safety and recognition of need for and safe use of fibrinolytics.

MANAGEMENT OF PATIENT IN ACUTE DECOMPENSATED HEART FAILURE

Management of patients presenting with acute decompensated heart failure (ADHF) includes vitals, SpO$_2$ monitoring and supplemental O$_2$ if needed, upright positioning, and cardiac monitoring. For patients presenting with respiratory distress or hypoxia already using oxygen, noninvasive ventilation should be attempted if there are no contraindications (suspected pending arrest, organ failure, upper airway obstruction, inability to clear or protect airway, low GSC, high risk for aspiration) and if intubation is not indicated. If intubation becomes necessary, etomidate is the induction agent of choice in RSI for ADHF. Immediate loop diuretics are indicated, noting that patients who have renal issues or have been on diuretics for long-term use may need to have higher dosages. Consider and treat or prepare receiving facility to treat causes of ADHF including- renal failure, sepsis, medications, HTN, ACS, valve regurgitation and new onset arrhythmias.

In patients with that don't know their type of heart failure or have known systolic heart failure (low ejection fraction), that present with severe ADHF with shock or pulmonary edema, use IV inotropes, such as dobutamine or milrinone, and transport patient to a facility with capabilities for mechanical support. If the patient reports history of diastolic HF and presents in shock, give IVF (after assessing for pulmonary edema) and an IV vasopressor.

TRANSCUTANEOUS PACING

Transcutaneous pacing is used temporarily to treat bradydysrhythmia that doesn't respond to medications and results in hemodynamic instability. The placement of pacing pads (large self-adhesive pads) and ECG leads varies somewhat according to the type of equipment, but usually one pacing pad (negative) is placed on the left chest, inferior to the clavicle, and the other (positive) on the left back, inferior to the scapula, so the heart is sandwiched between the two pads so that the myocardium is depolarized through the chest wall. Lead wires attach the pads to the monitor. The rate of pacing is usually set between 60 and 70 BPM. Current is increased slowly until capture occurs—a spiking followed by QRS sequence, then the current is readjusted downward if possible just to maintain capture. Both demand and fixed modes are available, but demand mode is preferred. Patients may require analgesia, especially if a higher current setting is needed.

ABDOMINAL AORTIC ANEURYSMS

An aneurysm occurs when a blood vessel expands beyond its normal size in a confined space. Aneurysms can lead to instant death, but patients with aneurysms can also be saved if the aneurysm is caught and treated in its early stages. A true aneurysm is one in which all three layers of the arterial wall are involved. These three layers are the adventia, the intima, and the media. Congenital malformations, high blood pressure, or infections can all lead to the development of true aneurysms. For many patients, they are not aware of an aortic aneurysm until there is a major problem. However, some patients have known aneurysms that are being monitored. The risk of rupture of the aneurysm increases with aneurysm diameter, and risk of rupture must be weighed with risk of surgery. Because of this, many CV surgeons don't choose to do aneurysm repair until the AAA is bigger than 5cm. 50% of patients with a rupture aneurysm will present with hypotension, severe pain, and a pulsating abdominal mass. Treating a patient with an AAA rupture, management is focused on maintaining hemodynamic status. If presenting with shock give IVF. For patients with blood pressures that are adequate, pain medications and prophylactic antiemetics are given. Note home meds, especially anticoagulants. Transfer to facility with CV surgery. For patients being transported between facilities for definitive care of a confirmed AAA, aggressive BP control is usually used with target SBPs often in the 100-120s, often with Esmolol.

BRADYCARDIA

Bradycardia – a condition in which a patient's heart beats at an abnormally slow rate of less than 60 beats per minute – is common among athletes and individuals who are physically fit, as their hearts are adequately able to pump blood efficiently at a lower rate than normal. Patients who use certain medications may also have an increased risk of developing bradycardia as a side effect of the medication(s). Sometimes, patients who have other medical conditions not related to their heart are more prone to developing the condition; these conditions include severe forms of liver disease; hypothyroidism, which is an abnormally low level of thyroid hormones; hypothermia, an abnormally low core body temperature; and brucellosis, an infectious disease that can cause fever, sweating, headaches, backaches, and physical lethargy in humans.

For new onset symptomatic bradycardia, after the airway is established, pulse oximetry, normal saline intravenously, and electrocardiographic monitoring, atropine is administered intravenously for adults at 0.5 mg push every 3–5 minutes (maximum 3 mg) If patient doesn't respond to atropine, dopamine or epinephrine drip may be tried prior to pacing. If the patient doesn't improve after 3 mg total atropine or 3rd degree heart block is noted, pace. Versed may be given if necessary for sedation and comfort.

FIRST DEGREE, WENCKEBACH, AND MOBITZ AV BLOCK

First degree AV block occurs when the atrial impulses are conducted through the AV node to the ventricles at a rate that is slower than normal. While the P and QRS are usually normal, the PR interval is >0.20 seconds, and the P:QRS ratio is 1:1. *Acute* first degree block is of more concern than chronic as it may be related to digoxin toxicity, β-blockers, amiodarone, myocardial infarction, hyperkalemia, or edema related to valvular surgery.

Second degree AV block, type I (Wenckebach): Each atrial impulse in a group of beats is conducted at a lengthened interval until one fails to conduct (the PR interval progressively increases), so there are more P waves than QRS complexes, but the QRS complex is usually of normal shape and duration. The sinus node functions at a regular rate, so the P-P interval is regular, but the R-R interval usually shortens with each impulse. The P:QRS ratio varies, such as 3:2, 4:3, 5:4.

Second degree AV block, type II (Mobitz): Only some of the atrial impulses are conducted unpredictably through the AV node to the ventricles, and the block always occurs below the AV node in the bundle of His, the bundle branches, or the Purkinje fibers. The PR intervals are the same if impulses are conducted, and QRS complex is usually widened. The P:QRS ratio varies 2:1, 3:1, and 4:1. Type II block is more dangerous than Type I because it may progress to complete AV block and may produce Stokes-Adams syncope.

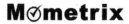

CLINICAL FACTORS ON WHICH TREATMENT OF ATRIAL FLUTTER OR ATRIAL FIBRILLATION IS BASED

Several clinical factors need to be taken into consideration when treating a patient with atrial flutter or atrial fibrillation. First, the patient should be classified as either clinically stable or clinically unstable. Second, the patient's cardiac functioning should be assessed, and a determination should be made as to whether the atrial flutter or fibrillation is impairing such functioning. Next, the absence or presence of Wolff-Parkinson-White syndrome should be determined; Wolff-Parkinson-White syndrome is characterized by electrical impulses arriving at the lower chambers of the heart, which are called the ventricles, too soon as a result of the presence of an extra conduction pathway in the heart. Finally, treatment should also be based in part on the length of time the flutter or fibrillation has been present.

Managing a-fib and a-flutter consists of controlling the ventricular rate, preventing emboli, converting to SR, and maintaining SR. For rate control calcium channel blockers and beta blockers are usually used. Electrical cardioversion or chemical conversion can be performed under the care of a physician. Of note, Ibutilide is the only FDA approved drug for chemical cardioversion of Aflutter.

ATRIAL TACHYCARDIA

Atrial tachycardia (AT) is classified into three categories based on the mechanisms that cause the condition; the categories are:

1. Intra-atrial reentry
2. Ectopic automaticity
3. Activity resulting from delayed after depolarization (DAD).

Patients with AT should be continually monitored for change in airway, breathing and circulation. Treatment includes:

- Diagnose the atrial rhythm to appropriately treat the underlying dysfunction.
- Identify and correct precipitating factors including hypokalemia and digitalis toxicity. In the stable, asymptomatic patient with AT, observation may be sufficient while investigating the cause.
- Vagal maneuvers can be tried and are most effective for focal AT.

Atrial tachycardia can result in supraventricular tachycardia, in which the ventricular rate becomes as rapid as the atrial rate. SVT often disguises the original dysrhythmia due to the rapid ventricular rate, therefore in order to differentiate the diagnosis, the ventricular rate must be slowed so that the P wave can be assessed. In stable adult patients for whom vagal maneuvers are unsuccessful in slowing the rate, IV beta blockers or calcium channel blockers may be used to control the rate. For a more aggressive option, known as chemical cardioversion, the patient should be placed on a cardiac monitor, and adenosine 6mg rapid IVP may be administered. If no change has occurred after two minutes, an additional 12 mg should be administered rapid IVP. Only two doses of adenosine are now recommended in ACLS protocol. Follow each dose with 20 cc rapid flush. (Patients with a transplanted heart, taking carbamazepine or dipyridamole or being given adenosine via central line should be given a 3 mg dose first, instead of 6 mg.) For children < 50 kg, 0.05 mg/kg rapid IVP. If the rhythm does not convert, increase by 0.05 mg/kg. This may be repeated until conversion or maximum dose of 0.3 mg/kg is reached. Rapid NS flushes must follow each dose. If hemodynamically instability occurs, electrical cardioversion is indicated.

POTENTIAL COMPLICATIONS WITH PERFORMING CARDIOVERSION

Cardioversion procedures are now routine procedures for patients with arrhythmias, but complications can arise. Patients can experience low blood pressure for several hours after a cardioversion has been performed, due to rhythm change, sedation and other factors.

For atrial fibrillation that is cardioverted, thromboembolism can occur, especially if the patient has had the AF for more than 48 hours and has not be on anticoagulant therapy. Thromboembolism can lead to stroke and pulmonary embolism.

Another complication includes risks incurred when the patient is given sedation. Most severe complications include breathing obstruction and aspiration leading to pneumonia. The patient could also have reactions to the medications used for cardioversion or sedation.

Other risks includes inducing other types of arrhythmias, especially bradycardias when the sinus node isn't functioning correctly, which then requires temporary pacing.

Occasionally heart tissue may be damaged due to repeated shocks, however this is uncommon. The pads used to provide the electric shock may cause pain, discomfort, and/or bruising at the placement site.

TRANSVENOUS PACEMAKERS

Transvenous pacemakers, comprised of a catheter with a lead at the end, may be used prophylactically or therapeutically on a temporary basis to treat a cardiac abnormality, especially bradycardia. The catheter is inserted through a vein at the femoral or neck area and attached to an external pulse generator. Clinical uses include:

- To treat persistent dysrhythmias not responsive to medications.
- To increase cardiac output with bradydysrhythmia by increasing rate.
- To decrease ventricular or supraventricular tachycardia by "overdrive" stimulation of contractions.
- To treat secondary heart block caused by myocardial infarction, ischemia, and drug toxicity.
- To improve cardiac output after cardiac surgery.
- To provide diagnostic information through electrophysiology studies, which induce dysrhythmias for purposes of evaluation.
- To provide pacing when a permanent pacemaker malfunctions.

Complications are similar to implanted pacemakers and include increased risk of pacemaker syndrome.

VF

Ventricular fibrillation (VF) is a rapid, very irregular ventricular rate >300 beats per minute with no atrial activity observable on the ECG, caused by disorganized electrical activity in the ventricles. The QRS complex is not recognizable as ECG shows irregular undulations. The causes are the same as for ventricular tachycardia (alcohol, caffeine, nicotine, underlying coronary disease), and VF may result if VT is not treated. VF may also result from an electrical shock or congenital disorder, such as Brugada syndrome. VF is accompanied by lack of palpable pulse, audible pulse, and respirations and is immediately life threatening without defibrillation. After emergency defibrillation, the cause should be identified and limited. Mortality is high if VF occurs as part of a myocardial infarction. Certain disorders of the heart can trigger VF, and the condition can also occur when the heart muscle does not receive an adequate supply of oxygen. Patients who have had a MI or congenital heart disease are at an increased risk of developing VF. Patients who have sustained heart trauma or undergone heart surgery are also at an increased risk for VF.

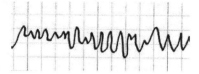

ECG OF PATIENT WITH PVT

Any recorded lead in an electrocardiogram (ECG) of a patient with polymorphic ventricular tachycardia (PVT) will display an unstable rhythm with a continuously varying QRS complex. The QT interval on an ECG of a patient with PVT can either be normal or prolonged; this interval assists with classifying the type of PVT present. PVT with a normal QT interval is an irregular rhythm that follows an acute coronary syndrome – such as cardiac arrest or unstable angina – or an episode of ischemia whereby the heart muscle does not receive enough blood and, subsequently, oxygen. PVT with a prolonged QT interval is known as torsades de pointes, which is a potentially deadly form of VT. The QRS complexes on an ECG of a patient with torsades de pointes swing up and down around the baseline in a disorganized manner.

INDICATIONS OF PERICARDIAL TAMPONADE

Pericardial tamponade occurs when fluid builds up in the membranes surrounding the heart, known as the pericardium. Upon physical examination, a patient with pericardial tamponade might exhibit signs of shock. Signs of shock can include loss of pigment in the skin, abnormally low blood pressure, excessive sweating, abnormal values for peripheral pulses, diminished capillary refill capacity, and/or shortness of breath. Another indicator of pericardial tamponade is the presence of Beck's triad, which is a medical condition comprised of three symptoms: 1) decrease in systolic pressure, 2) obscured heart sounds, and 3) enlargement of the jugular vein, a vein in the neck that transports blood from the head region to the heart.

SIGNS OF CARDIAC ARREST

Sudden cardiac arrest is the termination of cardiac movement and electrical activity, usually brought on by v-fib and v-tach. Without intervention it usually progresses to sudden cardiac death. Sudden cardiac arrest (SCA) may be preceded by warning signs but those signs may also be minimized and ignored by patients. A little more than 50% of patients had warning signs in the four weeks prior to arrest, with 80% having symptoms the hour before cardiac arrest. Chest pain and dyspnea are the two most commonly reported symptoms prior to SCA. Many patients with chest discomfort experience the sensation in the center of their chest; oftentimes, the pain or discomfort comes and goes, lasting several minutes each time. The discomfort is generally characterized as a tightening feeling, a feeling of squeezing in the chest, or pressure along the chest. Pain and discomfort in other areas of the body – including the back, the neck, either arm, the jaw, and/or the stomach – can also be signs, particularly when they are accompanied by chest pain. Shortness of breath and nausea or vomiting are additional signs of impending cardiac arrest. Once SCA happens the patient will be unresponsive, pulseless, with abnormal or absent breathing.

PERICARDIOCENTESIS

Blind (without ultrasound) pericardiocentesis is indicated with patient deterioration suspected to be from cardiac tamponade. All steps involved in an emergency pericardiocentesis must be exercised with extreme caution, as the environment make the procedure quite difficult. Patient should have IV, IVF running, ECG monitoring, airway and respiratory support. Position the patient at 30 to 45 degrees to bring the heart closest to chest wall, as this increases pooling in the heart.

Use aseptic technique, prep skin with chlorhexidine solution to the chest, drape area, wear PPE gear if at all possible. Anesthetize the insertion site and needle track in alert patient. Insert the pericardiocentesis needle, and advance it towards the pericardial sac, with continuous aspiration of the attached syringe. Upon reaching the pericardial sac with the needle, there is usually increased resistance and then a "pop", then fluid should be easily aspirated. If catheter-needle assembly is used, send a guide wire through the insertion site down towards the needle. Remove the needle, and replace it with a pericardial catheter, to drain the fluid from the sac. Hemodynamic improvement usually is the best indicator that pericardiocentesis was successful, as fluids draining can be from other sites or due to cardiac puncture. The site for a blind pericardiocentesis has typically been subxiphoid, however current studies show that the left parasternal and apical approaches yield superior results.

MANAGEMENT OF SUSPECTED AORTIC DISSECTION

An aortic dissection is life threatening with a mortality rate of 27%. Aortic dissections often arise in a preexisting aneurysm with 65% in the ascending, 10% in the arch, and 20% in the descending aorta. Symptoms include abrupt, acute chest pain, although patients with a congenital defect (Marfan's disease) may lack pain. Symptoms may mimic a myocardial infarction, but ECG indications of an MI are missing. Patients may exhibit JVD, pulsus paradoxus, and muffled cardiac sounds if the dissection results in cardiac tamponade. BP may be increased or decreased, depending on the type of dissection. One indication of aortic dissection is blood pressure difference between right and left arms of greater than 20 mmHg. Patients may exhibit both neurologic and respiratory impairments. Interventions include ECG and cardiac monitoring, intubation/ventilation if unstable, insertion of two large-bore IV lines, and administration of morphine for pain. If BP is elevated, propranolol or another beta-blocker may be given to decrease BP and pulse rate. If BP remains high, nitroprusside sodium may be administered.

ACUTE EXACERBATION OF CONGESTIVE HEART FAILURE

An acute exacerbation of congestive heart failure may involve right-sided or left-sided failure although most patients exhibit signs of both. LV dysfunction is most common.

- Right failure: Generalized edema, hepatic congestion, anorexia, nausea, and ascites.
- Left failure: Low cardiac output, increased pulmonary venous pressure with pronounced dyspnea.

Most patients will complain of orthopnea, paroxysmal nocturnal dyspnea, and dyspnea at rest as condition deteriorates. If CHF is related to MI or endocarditis with valvular regurgitation, the patient will have pulmonary edema. Patients with intermittent ischemia may have episodic symptoms. Initial treatment for most patients with severe CHF is oxygen to relieve acute dyspnea, a loop diuretic (such as furosemide) and an ACE inhibitor (such as captopril), position of comfort (head elevated), and cardiac monitoring. Because ACE inhibitors may induce hypotension, a low initial dose should be administered. Severely hypotensive patients may require dobutamine if nonresponsive to other treatments.

HYPERTENSIVE CRISIS

Hypertensive crisis (AKA malignant hypertension) is marked elevation in blood pressure than can cause severe organ damage if left untreated. Causes include encephalopathy, intracranial hemorrhage, aortic dissection, eclampsia, and heart failure. Classifications:

- Hypertensive emergency: Acute hypertension, usually >120 mmHg diastolic, must be treated immediately to lower blood pressure in order to prevent damage to vital organs, such as the heart, brain, or kidneys.
- Hypertensive urgency: Acute hypertension must be treated within a few hours but the vital organs are not in immediate danger. Blood pressure is lowered more slowly to avoid hypotension, ischemia of vital organs, or failure of autoregulation with 1/3 reduction in 6 hours.

Symptoms include headache, dizziness, dyspnea, weakness, visual disturbances, anxiety, chest pain (atypical), heart failure, acute coronary syndrome, and stroke. Prehospital: Severe symptoms require rapid transport. Interventions include airway support/ventilation with oxygen supplementation, IV line access and advanced life support as needed. Sodium nitroprusside is given for fast-acting vasodilation. Patients with severe dyspnea and pulmonary edema may need CPAP.

ARTERIAL LINE

Arterial lines are used for continuous BP monitoring, frequent blood sampling, and ABGs. Arterial lines are inserted into the radial (preferred) or femoral artery. Before radial insertion, the CRFN should conduct the Allen test to ensure adequate circulation to the hand. Contraindications include coagulopathy, inadequate circulation, Raynaud's syndrome and Buerger disease. The most common catheter is the 7 Fr 15 or 20 cm triple lumen. For insertion, the patient should be placed in supine position with wrist in a supported, dorsiflexed (30-45°) position with palm up. Lidocaine 1% should be injected for conscious patients. A catheter-over-needle or catheter-over-wire technique may be utilized with the needle inserted at a 30° to 45° angle. (If utilizing the catheter-over-wire technique, a small nick with a scalpel at the insertion site is needed to allow passage of the catheter.) Once the catheter is in place, the catheter must be secured with a suture or tape, site monitored carefully, and circulation in the hand assessed frequently.

CARE AND ASSESSMENT OF CENTRAL LINES BEFORE AND DURING TRANSPORT

Central lines are central venous access devices (CVD) inserted for long-term IV therapy. Types include peripherally inserted central catheters (PICC), non-tunneled percutaneous central venous catheters, tunneled central venous catheters, and implanted subcutaneous ports. The PICC line is inserted into a lower arm vein while the others are inserted into veins in the right upper chest or neck with the tips of all types in the superior vena cava. The most common complication is infection. Before transport, the CFRN should assess the type of CVAD, manufacturer's directions (if available), schedules for treatments (IVs, blood products, medications) or testing, patient skin turgor, and condition of skin about insertion site for signs of infiltration, extravasation, and/or infection. The CRFN should determine if any lumen needs flushing, check all connection points, and assess length of catheter. During transfer and transport, the CFRN should protect the CVAD to prevent dislodgement or catheter damage by using a catheter stabilization device or looping and taping securely.

MONITORING CENTRAL VENOUS PRESSURE

Central venous pressure (CVP) is monitored through a central venous catheter with a pressure monitoring device attached to the distal port and threaded into one of the major vessels with the tip resting in the superior vena cava. The transducer should be placed at the midaxillary line, fourth intercostal space. CVP is the pressure in the superior vena cava or right atrium related to either volume or compliance. The normal CVP ranges from 2 to 6 mmHg. If the CVP increases to greater than 6 mmHg, this may indicate hypervolemia (such as may occur with renal failure), right-sided heart failure (decreased cardiac output and stroke volume), pulmonary artery stenosis, or positive pressure breathing (Valsalva maneuver). If the pressure falls below 2 mmHg, it most often represents hypovolemia, which may result from dehydration, blood loss, diarrhea, vomiting, and excessive diuresis. CVP may also decrease with negative pressure breathing.

SWAN-GANZ CATHETERIZATION

Swan-Ganz catheterization is a procedure whereby a catheter is passed into the right side of a patient's heart to monitor heart functioning and to examine blood flow. Normal diastolic pressure of the pulmonary artery ranges from zero to eight millimeters of mercury (mmHg); normal pulmonary artery systolic pressure is 15 to 30 mmHg. The mean pulmonary artery pressure is 12 mmHg. Pulmonary capillary wedge pressure normally ranges from five to 15 mmHg, and the normal range for right atrial pressure is zero to eight mmHg. If the monitor calculates cardiac output, normal ranges are 4-8 L/min and normal cardiac index is 2.5 to 4.2 L/min/m². However, before interfacility transfer, note that numbers that have been normal for that patient this admission to compare with any changes during flight, as these patients may not have normal numbers.

After transferring patient to aircraft, connect transducers to monitor (if transport monitor isn't compatible). Rezero the transducers. Make sure to release any extra air in the fluid bag of the pressure bag to avoid expansion during flight. Frequently monitor pressure of bag when flying (maintain 300 mm Hg).

PHENYLEPHRINE HYDROCHLORIDE

Phenylephrine hydrochloride (Neo-synephrine®), a vasoconstrictor/alpha adrenergic agent (pregnancy Category C), treats hypotension (including drug-induced). IV administration has immediate onset and 15-20-minute duration. IM/SC administration has 10-15 minute onset and 0.5-2-hour duration. Dosage:

- Mild to moderate hypotension: Adult— IV: 0.1-0.5 mg and repeat in 10 to 15 minutes as needed; 1 to 10 mg IM/SC: first dose of ≤5 mg and repeat in 1 to 2 hours if needed. Pediatric—0.1 mg/kg. IM/SC and repeat in 1 to 2 hours if needed.
- Severe hypotension/shock: Adult—10 mg in 250-500 mL D₅W or NS. Initially at 100-180 mcg/minute and decreased to 40-60 mcg/minute after BP stabilizes.
- Paroxysmal SVT: Adult—Initially 0.5mg rapid IV infusion with increase in 0.1 to 0.2 mg dosages to maximum single dose of 1 mg.

Monitor ECG, vital signs, urinary output, and circulation to limbs (color, temperature). Follow protocol or for patients with history of hypertension, maintain BP at 30-40 mmHg below baseline, and for patients with no history of hypertension, maintain systolic BP at 80-100 mmHg.

NOREPINEPHRINE BITARTRATE

Norepinephrine bitartrate (Levophed®) is a vasopressor/direct-acting adrenergic agent (pregnancy Category C) used to treat acute hypotension, especially hypotension associated with cardiogenic or septic shock. The drug should only be administered intravenously in D₅W or D₅NS solution, usually through a central venous catheter or large vein. The initial dose is 8 to 12 mcg/min and it can then be titrated to an average maintenance dose of 2 to 4 mcg/min. For patients with history of hypertension, maintain BP at 40 mmHg below baseline, and for patients with no history of hypertension, maintain systolic BP at 80 to 100 mmHg. The patient should have continuous monitoring with vital signs assessed every 2 minutes until stable and then every 5 minutes. Monitor ECG, vital signs, urinary output, and circulation to limbs (color, temperature). Monitor site for signs of extravasation or blanching, which is treated by stopping the infusion, aspirating (but not flushing) IV, removing IV, elevating extremity and then injecting area with phentolamine diluted in 10 to 15 ml NS, to prevent tissue necrosis.

DOPAMINE

Dopamine, a vasopressor/adrenergic agonist (pregnancy Category C), is used to treat hemodynamic instability caused by shock or heart failure in adults and children. It is administered intravenously in D_5W, NS, D_5W in NS, 0.45% saline, or Lactated Ringer's through a central line or large vein to prevent extravasation. Dosage for adults and children initially is 2 to 5 mcg/kg/min. The drug is titrated by 1 to 4 mcg/kg/min every 10 to 30 minutes. If the patient is severely ill, the maximum initial dosage of 5 mcg/kg/min should be used and titrated by adding 5 to 10 mcg/kg/min to a maximum of 20 to 50 mcg/kg/min. If the patient has vascular occlusive disease, the initial dosage should begin with 1 mcg/kg/min. Monitor ECG, vital signs, urinary output, and circulation to limbs (color, temperature). Avoid administering a bolus of the drug. Monitor site for signs of extravasation or blanching, which is treated by stopping infusion and infiltrating area with phentolamine diluted in 10 to 15 ml NS, to prevent tissue necrosis.

CARING FOR PATIENT WITH VAD

A ventricular assist device (VAD) is a small pump implanted into the patient's chest or abdomen. The left ventricular assist device, or LVAD (the most common type of VAD), takes blood from the left ventricle through an inflow tube to the pump, which pumps it though an outflow tube to the aorta where it circulates. A driveline (cable) connects the implanted device to a computerized control unit outside of the body. The control unit is attached by additional cables to a power module or to 2 lithium battery packs and carried in a patient pack or special vest. LVADs are non-pulsatile, so a peripheral pulse is not palpable. Batteries must be changed one at a time (the pair last 10-12 hours). LVADs have alarm systems with symbols or messages to describe problems, such as disconnected cables or hypovolemia. INR target varies according to manufacturer, and is usually 2-3. Complications include right HF, arrhythmias, thrombus, stroke, bleeding, infection, hypovolemia, and device malfunction. Patients may not have obvious signs initially of arrhythmias (such as VFib), but they must be treated promptly to prevent organ failure.

IABP

Intraaortic Balloon Counterpulsation (IABC, also known as IABPs) is a cardiac assist device used to treat patients with cardiogenic shock or severe perfusion issues. The primary purpose of an IABP is to increase the myocardial oxygen supply while decreasing the myocardial oxygen demand. The balloon needs to be inflated and deflated according to the patient's cardiac cycle; if the inflation and deflation are not timed correctly, the issue of myocardial oxygen supply vs demand will not be resolved. In addition to improper balloon placement, other complications can occur. Limb ischemia, a condition in which the arteries become obstructed and subsequently decrease the flow of blood to the patient's extremities, is one of the most common complications. Other complications can include infection, hemorrhage, circulatory problems, and aortic rupture. The CFRN should assess the IABP insertion site and distal limb prior to transporting a patient with an IABP and note adequate perfusion. The site of insertion should be noted for hematoma, bleeding or s/s of infection. If hematoma is present, area should be outlined and assessed frequently for growth. New sharp back or groin pain, hypotension, tachycardia, bruises to abdomen and flank could indicate retroperitoneal bleeding, a very severe complication. If a patient with an IABP has cardiac arrest, most pump manufacturers recommend switching from ECG trigger to AP trigger, due to loss of ECG rhythm. The pump doesn't have to be disconnected during defibrillation.

INDUCED HYPOTHERMIA

Induced hypothermia (usually for 12 to 24 hours) maintains body temperature at a level lower than normal in order to provide neuroprotection following a period in which circulation to the brain was inadequate, such as after cardiac arrest. Induced hypothermia may also be used with some surgical procedures. Mild hypothermia is cooling the body to 32° to 35° C.; moderate hypothermia is 28° to 32° C; and deep hypothermia is <28° C. (Some studies suggest that cooling below 32° C has no advantage.) Management includes careful temperature monitoring and recording of temperature every hour. Vasopressors may be needed if systolic BP falls below 90 mmHg or MAP above 75 mmHg. Urinary output should be monitored and the physician should be alerted if output falls above 200 mL or below 30 mL for 2 consecutive hours. An NMBA (such as vecuronium) is used to prevent shivering in conjunction with sedation (such as midazolam). Pupillary reactions should be checked at least every hour.

ASSESSING FOR UPPER RESPIRATORY DISTRESS

A patient who is taking more breaths per minute than normal may be having difficulty breathing and/or may now have an adequate supply of oxygen. Additionally, patients who are not getting enough oxygen may display a bluish tint to their lips – either around the mouth or on the inside of the lips. Skin that looks pale or gray in tone may also indicate a lack of oxygen. Oftentimes, patients produce a grunting noise when they are having trouble breathing. This grunting noise is apparent when the patient exhales. The noise is caused by the body attempting to keep the lungs filled with air. When a patient's nostrils flare when he/she breathes, it may indicate that the patient is exerting more effort than usual to breathe, which may in turn signify upper respiratory distress. Sweating, particularly along the forehead, and wheezing are also indicators of upper respiratory problems.

QUESTIONS TO ASK PATIENTS HAVING DIFFICULTY BREATHING

The following are the types of questions to ask a patient presenting with breathing difficulties:

- How long have you been having trouble breathing?
- Did your breathing difficulties come on suddenly?
- Do you have additional symptoms or other medical conditions?
- In what position are your breathing difficulties at their worst?
- Does physical activity make it even more difficult for you to breathe?
- Are you able to breathe easier when you are not exerting yourself?
- Do you feel like you are short of breath?
- Do you have episodes of breathing difficulty or is the difficulty continuous?
- If you have episodes of breathing difficulty, how long does each episode last?
- Have you been exposed to anything or ingested anything to which you are allergic?
- Can you hear any abnormal sounds each time you breathe?
- Do your breathing difficulties prevent you from sleeping?
- Do your breathing difficulties awaken you when you are asleep?

INSPECTION AND PALPATION OF THE CHEST

Inspection of the chest is performed, in part, to determine a patient's respiratory rate. The rate can be determined by counting the number of breaths the patient takes in a minute through observing his/her chest rise and fall. A rate of 12 breaths per minute is considered normal respiration for adults. Inspection of the chest can provide additional information about irregular or abnormal patterns of breathing as well as breathing difficulties. The examiner should also observe the patient's chest for asymmetry and/or deformity during the inspection process. During palpation of the chest, the examiner should assess any areas of tenderness. Similar to the inspection process, palpation of the chest should include an assessment of deformities uncovered during the process. A diminished vibration level in the chest when a patient speaks may indicate a potentially serious lung condition or other medical complication.

NORMAL AND ABNORMAL BREATH SOUNDS

Vesicular	Normal low-pitched sound over lung bases and most lung fields.
Broncho-vesicular	Medium-pitched sound heard over main bronchi. Duration the same in expiration and inspiration.
Bronchial	Normal high-pitched loud sound heard over trachea. Expiratory sound is as long or longer than inspiratory. Abnormal if heard over lung bases.
Rales (crackles)	High-pitched crackles usually heard at end of expiration in lung bases indicating fluid in the alveoli. May be fine or coarse.
Rhonchi	Deep rumbling sound may be high-pitched and sibilant (whistling) or low-pitched and sonorous (snoring) caused by constricted airways or large amounts of secretions in airways. More pronounced on expiration.
Wheezes	High or low-pitched whistling or musical sounds most pronounced on expiration. Often indicate asthma or foreign body obstruction.
Stridor	Crowing sound caused by inflammation and swelling or larynx and trachea. Common finding in croup (associated with cough).
Grunts	Indicates respiratory distress in newborn.
Friction rub	Grating sound heard over area of lungs where pleura are inflamed.

PERCUSSION OF THE CHEST

To percuss a patient's chest, the examiner should place one of his/her middle fingers upon the chest so that the distal interphalangeal joint lies firmly against the chest. Using the tip of his/her opposite middle finger, the examiner should use a flicking motion to strike the finger that is placed against the patient's chest. The resulting sound(s) should be documented; the sound(s) should be recorded as normal, dull, or hyperresonant. Dull sounds resulting from chest percussion may indicate pleural effusion – fluid accumulation in the pleural space – or lung consolidation – hardening or swelling of lung tissue. Exaggerated resonance can indicate conditions such as pneumothorax – air accumulation in the pleural space – or pulmonary diseases such as emphysema.

PP

During respiration, variation in a patient's pulse occurs as a normal process. Typically, a patient's pulse is weaker during inhalation and stronger when the patient exhales. Pulsus paradoxus (PP) is characterized by an abnormal pulse variation during respiration. Such variation can be a sign of a more serious medical condition such as chronic obstructive pulmonary disease (COPD) or asthma. A blood pressure cuff and stethoscope are generally used to measure PP. By examining the patient's systolic blood pressure variation with respiration, PP can either be indicated or ruled out. PP is indicated when a reduction in systolic pressure upon inspiration is greater than 10 millimeters of mercury (mmHg), as normal systolic blood pressure variation with respiration is 10 mmHg.

NEEDLE DECOMPRESSION

Needle decompression, also referred to as needle thoracostomy, and is indicated for hemodynamically unstable patients with a suspected tension pneumothorax. A needle decompression is performed by inserting a large needle into intercostal space along the patient's midclavicular plane. The purpose of the needle insertion is to release the pressure that has built up in the patient's chest as a result of the trapped air. Most aircrafts have readily available kits with 14 or 16 gauge angiocatheters in them. The angiocatheter is placed on the affected side, third intercostal space, and midclavicular. This allows for immediate decompression. The needle is withdrawn and the cath remains in place, open to air. Usually there is rush of air on placement that indicates there is in fact a tension pneumo, as well as improvement in vital signs post placement. The small catheters are prone to kinks and small so they may not be able to completely remove the pneumo, so when stabilized and able, place a standard chest tube.

ASSESSMENT OF DIALYSIS SITES FOR PATIENTS WITH ESRD

When assessing dialysis sites (usually AV fistula or graft) for patients with ESRD, the CFRN should assess the skin to determine if it appears normal and without swelling, erythema, or discharge indicative of infection. The site should be palpated for indications of swelling (aneurysm/pseudoaneurysm), thrombosis, or stenosis. A thrill should be felt only at the arterial anastomosis; a marked thrill elsewhere may indicate stenosis. The bruit should be low pitched and continuous on auscultation. A high-pitched discontinuous bruit may indicate stenosis. The pulse should be soft and easy to compress. Circulation should also be assessed in the extremity distal to the fistula or graft. Swelling or lack of pulse many indicate obstruction. The dialysis access site and the extremity containing the dialysis access site should not be used for IVs, blood draws, or blood pressure readings. Because patients may have had previous access sites and may have extensive scarring, finding a vein to use can be challenging. The patient may be able to provide guidance.

MEDICATION CAUTIONS/CONSIDERATIONS IN PATIENTS WITH ESRD

Because patients with end-stage-renal disease (ESRD) are unable to adequately remove body fluids through urination, intravenous fluids should be restricted in these patients, although a fluid bolus may be needed for hypovolemia or hypotension. If a patient is in a state of fluid overload already (such as right before a scheduled hemodialysis treatment), IV fluids may result in pulmonary edema. The patient's residual urinary output (if any) should be determined, and the dosage of some common drugs excreted through the kidneys reduced to avoid toxicity or overdose. Some medications, such as loop diuretics, may be ineffective if a patient has no urinary output. Many drugs are excreted by the kidneys (antibiotics, beta-blockers, lithium, digoxin, and ranitidine) and must be administered with caution. If a patient is receiving hemodialysis, this process may decrease serum levels of some medications, such as anticonvulsants, especially immediately after dialysis, so dosages may need to be increased.

ASSESSING AND TREATING DIALYSIS PATIENTS
HYPOTENSION AND DEHYDRATION

Hypotension is a common problem associated with hemodialysis because up to 400 mL of blood is outside of the body during the process and excess fluid is removed rapidly. Hypotension can also result from eating during hemodialysis. Symptoms include nausea and vomiting, dizziness, impaired perfusion, confusion, chest pain, seizures, and arrhythmias. Hypotension during treatment is usually treated with a bolus of fluid and lowering the patient's head. If hypotension persists, the patient may require further fluid resuscitation and supportive care.

Dehydration can occur from dialysis removing too much body fluid, toxin buildup, inadequate fluid intake, or excessive loss of body fluids, such as may occur with strenuous exercise or exposure to high environmental temperatures, especially shortly after dialysis. Patients are usually limited to fluid intake of 32 to 50 ounces daily, depending on age, size, and activity level. Symptoms include nausea, tachycardia, thirst, dry mouth, itching, and anxiety. Treatment includes careful administration of IV fluids and treatment of hypernatremia.

HYPERKALEMIA AND BLEEDING

Hyperkalemia (>5.5 mEq/L with a critical value >6.5 mEq/L) is common in dialysis patients and can be related to constipation and excessive intake of potassium. Symptoms include ventricular arrhythmias leading to cardiac arrest, weakness, hyperreflexia, diarrhea, and confusion. Treatment includes ECG monitoring, calcium carbonate (to decrease cardiac abnormalities), sodium bicarbonate, insulin, and hypertonic dextrose (to temporarily shift potassium into cells), sodium polystyrene sulfonate (Kayexalate®) retention enema (to decrease potassium), and a dialysis treatment.

Bleeding may result from the heparin required for hemodialysis and thrombocytopenia. Patients may develop bruising, bleeding of gums, nosebleeds, and prolonged bleeding after removal of needles. Patients are at risk for internal bleeding (GI, intracranial). Outflow stenosis of the AV shunt may also cause prolonged bleeding after needle removal, so the shunt should be carefully assessed. Treatment depends on the severity of bleeding and ranges from applying pressure to transfusions to heparin antidote (protamine sulfate1%).

REFLEX RESPONSES

Primitive reflexes are typically present only in infants; adults who exhibit primitive reflexes have typically suffered from stroke or some type of damage to the brain. Primitive reflexes include such reflexes as grasping, which occurs when an infant closes his/her hand around an adult's finger, and rooting, which is characterized by an infant turning his/her head and making a sucking motion in response to cheek stroking. Superficial reflexes include the abdominal, anal, conjunctival, corneal, cremasteric, and plantar reflexes. When assessed, superficial reflexes can support or refute the functioning of cutaneous innervation as well as the motor functioning of the corresponding part of the reflex being assessed. Deep tendon reflexes, which include the ankle, biceps, brachioradialis, patellar, and triceps, are reflexes of the tendons that attach the muscles located next to bones to the bones themselves.

SUPERFICIAL REFLEXES

When the abdominal reflex is tested by stimulating the skin covering the abdomen, the muscles of the abdominal wall should contract. Irritating a patient's perianal skin, the skin around the opening of the rectum, will cause the anal sphincter to contract if the anal reflex is intact. A patient's eyelid will close when the conjunctiva is touched if his/her conjunctival reflex is working. Additionally, a patient will blink when the cornea is stimulated if his/her corneal reflex is intact; this reflex is also known as the blink reflex. The cremasteric reflex is specific to males; when this reflex is functioning, the cremaster muscle will contract and pull up the patient's scrotum and testis upon stimulation of the front and inner thigh. The plantar reflex can be tested by stroking the outer surface of the soles of a patient's feet, which should cause his/her toes to flex.

DEEP TENDON REFLEXES

The biceps reflex can be observed when the examiner places his/her thumb over the patient's biceps tendon at the elbow, strikes his/her thumb with a reflex hammer, and watches for movement in the patient's arm. The triceps reflex can be observed when the examiner holds the patient's upper arm in one hand and strikes the triceps tendon, located on the back side of the arm just above the elbow, with a reflex hammer. With the patient's lower arm hanging in a relaxed position, it should swing away from the patient's body in response to the hammer strikes. With the patient's arm resting in his/her lap, the brachioradialis reflex can be observed by striking the brachioradialis tendon – located in approximately the middle of the superior side of the patient's lower arm – with a reflex hammer.

The ankle reflex, which is sometimes referred to as the Achilles reflex, can be observed by holding the patient's foot in a dorsiflexed position – whereby the foot is bent backwards towards the patient – and tapping the Achilles tendon, which connects the heel bone and the calf muscle, with a reflex hammer. The patellar reflex, which is also known as the knee jerk reflex, is best observed while the patient is in a seated position with his/her legs hanging over the edge of the examining surface. When the patellar tendon – located just at the bottom of the kneecap on the front side of the patient's knee – is struck with a reflex hammer, the patient's lower leg should extend outward at the knee, making a small kicking motion.

CLONUS

Clonus can be described as a series of rapid muscle contractions that occur involuntarily when a muscle is stretched. Clonus can indicate the presence of certain neurological abnormalities and is often associated with spinal cord injuries, stroke, and multiple sclerosis. The ankles are one of the most common areas for clonus to be present; as such, an ankle clonus test is often performed to assess for clonus. The test is performed by gently bending the patient's foot backwards – dorsiflexing the foot – towards him/her. Rapid muscle contractions will persist while the patient's foot is in a dorsiflexed position if clonus is present.

STATUS EPILEPTICUS

Status epilepticus (SE) is usually generalized tonic-clonic seizures that are characterized by a series of seizures with intervening time too short for regaining of consciousness. The constant assault and periods of apnea can lead to exhaustion, respiratory failure with hypoxemia and hypercapnia, cardiac failure, and death.

Causes	Treatment
Uncontrolled epilepsy or non-compliance with anticonvulsants. Infections, such as encephalitis. Encephalopathy or stroke. Drug toxicity (isoniazid). Brain trauma. Neoplasms. Metabolic disorders.	Seizure precautions to keep patient safe. IV access for benzos and RSI meds if needed. Secure airway and provided associated supportive care. Anticonvulsants beginning with fast-acting benzodiazepines, usually lorazepam 0.1 mg/kg IV at a rate of 2 mg/min. Allow 1-2 minutes after dose has been given to assess if seizures continue. If they continue, subsequent doses of Ativan can be given, monitoring sedative effects and bp. Diazepam can be given instead of lorazepam- 0.2 mg/kg IV.

NUCHAL RIGIDITY AND MENINGITIS

Nuchal rigidity is a condition whereby a patient is not able to flex his/her head as a result of the neck muscles being rigid, or stiff. The condition can be an indicator of a problem with or irritation to the meninges, which are the membranes that surround the patient's central nervous system. Nuchal rigidity is associated with bacterial meningitis but is not exclusive to that process.

Patients with bacterial meningitis may exhibit signs to help support the diagnosis. While the following are not universally present, they are specific to meningitis and are rarely positive with other disorders:

- Kernig's sign: Flex each hip and then try to straighten the knee while the hip is flexed. Spasm of the hamstrings makes this painful and difficult with meningitis.
- Brudzinski sign: With the patient lying supine, flex the neck by pulling head toward chest. The neck stiffness causes the hips and knees to pull up into a flexed position with meningitis.

Jolt accentuation maneuver: (Used if nuchal rigidity is not present.) Ask patient to rapidly move his/her head from side to side horizontally. Increase in headache is positive for meningitis.

HYPOGLYCEMIA AND HYPERGLYCEMIA

Hypoglycemia occurs when a patient's serum glucose level drops too low to sustain the patient's activities. Symptoms of hypoglycemia can include trembling or feeling shaky, extreme hunger, feeling weak, difficulty communicating effectively, heart palpitations, sweating. Untreated theses can lead to acute hypoglycemia where the patient has a decrease in LOC, respiratory distress, tachycardia, etc.

Hyperglycemia is elevation of serum glucose ≥ 180 mg/dL although symptoms may not be evident until the level reaches ≥ 270 mg/dL. The most common cause is diabetes mellitus (associated with decreased levels of insulin), but elevations of glucose may also be related to chronic pancreatitis, acromegaly, Cushing's syndrome, and adverse reactions to drugs, such as furosemide, glucocorticoids, growth hormone, oral contraceptives, and thiazides. Symptoms of hyperglycemia may include frequent feelings of hunger and/or thirst and a frequent need to urinate. Although they are not the most common symptoms, dry mouth, weight loss, fatigue, blurred vision, and recurrent infections such as ear infections may also be indicators of hyperglycemia.

MANAGING SYMPTOMS OF HYPOGLYCEMIA

Acute hypoglycemia (hyperinsulinism) may result from pancreatic islet tumors or hyperplasia, increasing insulin production, or from the use of insulin to control diabetes mellitus. Hyperinsulinism can cause damage to the central nervous and cardiopulmonary systems, interfering with functioning of the brain and causing neurological impairment.

Causes may include:

- Genetic defects in chromosome 11 (short arm).
- Severe infections, such as Gram-negative sepsis, endotoxic shock.
- Toxic ingestion of alcohol or drugs, such as salicylates.

- Too much insulin for body needs.
- Too little food or excessive exercise.

Symptoms	Treatment
Blood glucose <50-60 mg/dL. Central nervous system: seizures, altered consciousness, lethargy, and poor feeding with vomiting, myoclonus, respiratory distress, diaphoresis, hypothermia, and cyanosis. Adrenergic system: diaphoresis, tremor, tachycardia, palpitation, hunger, and anxiety.	Glucose/Glucagon administration to elevate blood glucose levels. Careful monitoring. Identifying meds patient is on that could be contributing to hypoglycemia. Identifying infection/toxic ingestions Identifying reasons for too little caloric intake

DKA

Diabetic ketoacidosis most often occurs because of non-adherence to diet and insulin requirements or in previously undiagnosed diabetics. Onset is usually rapid, occurring within a few days. Because insulin is not available to metabolize glucose, lipolysis occurs with glycerol in fat cells and is converted to ketone bodies. Excess ketones are excreted through the kidneys (ketonuria) or exhalations. Symptoms include ketoacidosis (serum ketones >5 mEq/L, pH <7.3, bicarbonate < 15 mEq/L), nausea and vomiting, Kussmaul respirations (hyperventilation with "ketone" breath), polyuria, polydipsia, dehydration (up to deficit of 6L), hypokalemia with cardiac arrhythmias, hyperglycemia (>300 mg/dL), confusion, and disorientation. Prehospital: Monitor glucose level, assess skin turgor and level of consciousness, obtain 12-lead ECG and continuous cardiac monitoring, provide O_2 to maintain oxygen saturation of 92-96%, provide IV access and NS IV up to 3 L in first hour. Insulin is usually withheld until potassium level is obtained and dehydration is reversed. Sodium bicarbonate may be administered if seizures occur.

DIABETES INSIPIDUS

Diabetes insipidus (DI) may be central (characterized by decreased levels of antidiuretic hormone [ADH]), or nephrogenic (characterized by renal ADH resistance). DI may be also psychogenic from fluid intake >5L day. Central DI, transient or permanent, is most common in critical care, especially with traumatic brain injury, surgery in the area of the pituitary or hypothalamus, brain tumors, and encephalitis/meningitis. Primary symptoms of DI are polydipsia and polyuria (3 to 20 L output daily). Symptoms include dry skin, fatigue, and hair loss. If unable to drink adequate fluids, patients may become dehydrated and develop hypernatremia. With hypernatremia, the patient should receive D_5W IV at 500-750 mL per hour to decrease Na levels by 0.5 mEq/L per hour. The drug of choice for central DI is desmopressin: intranasal 10-40 mcg daily in one or divided doses; oral 0.1-1.2 in divided doses 2-3 times daily; IV/SC 2-4 mcg daily in divided doses. Administering desmopressin immediately before transport may delay the need to urinate if the patient is not catheterized.

NORMAL COAGULATION

Coagulation is the process whereby blood turns from a liquid to a solid and forms clots. In a normal coagulation process, a substance known as fibrin is formed through blood clotting factors involved in an elaborate chemical process. Ultimately, the fibrin assists with the formation of a clot, which stops the bleeding. During the typical coagulation process, the patient's blood vessels constrict when bleeding occurs. A platelet plug begins to control the bleeding, and then a fibrin clot develops to eventually stop the bleeding altogether. This process does not occur normally in patients who have coagulation disorders or deficiencies, which can lead to additional illnesses or medical complications.

THROMBOCYTOPENIA

Thrombocytopenia is a condition characterized by a deficient number of platelets in the blood, which are cells that assist with clotting. Patients can develop a low platelet count in their bone marrow as one of the causes of thrombocytopenia. Aplastic anemia, bone marrow cancer and some bone marrow infections, and certain medications – although quite rare – can lead to an insufficient platelet count in a patient's bone marrow. Intravascular thrombocytopenia can occur when platelets break down in a patient's bloodstream, resulting in a deficiency. Additionally, a patient's spleen or liver can experience a break down in platelet level, which is referred to as extravascular thrombocytopenia.

ANEMIA, LEUKOPENIA, AND THROMBOCYTOPENIA

Anemia is a condition whereby a patient has a deficiency of red blood cells in his/her blood. Red blood cells transport oxygen to tissue; consequently, anemia results in an inadequate oxygen supply to a patient's tissue. The condition can indicate potentially serious illnesses. A low white blood cell count characterizes the condition known as leukopenia. White blood cells primarily function to fight infection. While a moderate decrease in white blood cells may not indicate a serious illness, a significantly low white blood cell count – a count lower than 2,500 cells per microliter – can significantly increase a patient's likelihood of developing a serious infection. Thrombocytopenia is a condition whereby a patient has a deficient number of platelets in his/her blood. As an adequate platelet supply is essential for normal blood clotting, patients with thrombocytopenia often experience complications with clotting.

PREHOSPITAL MANAGEMENT OF ACUTE EXACERBATION OF CHRONIC THROMBOCYTOPENIA, ITP, OR TTP

Chronic thrombocytopenia (CT) is a condition in which a patient's platelet count is chronically below normal, which ranges from 150,000 to 450,000. CT may result from decreased platelet production (chronic alcoholism, bone marrow failure, and vitamin B-12/folate deficiency), increased platelet consumption (mechanical destruction, preeclampsia, DIC, HIT, ITP), and sequestration (dilutional, gestational, hepatic disease, pulmonary embolism). Immune thrombocytic purpura (ITP) results in impairment of the clotting mechanism because of inadequate numbers of platelets, resulting in increased bruising and bleeding. Thrombotic thrombocytopenia purpura (TTP), on the other hand, results in clotting in small vessels because of increased platelet aggregation. This, in turn, results in decreased circulating platelets and increased risk of bruising and bleeding. Acute exacerbation of any type of thrombocytopenia, especially when platelet count falls to ≤20,000, can result in hemorrhage. Prehospital management includes controlling any bleeding, supportive care, and oxygen if blood loss has been significant. Patients with CT/ITP may require corticosteroids, IVIg or RhIG, and platelet transfusions with severe hemorrhage. Patients with TTP may require plasma exchange.

PV

Polycythemia vera (PV) is a condition characterized by increased blood cell production; patients with PV primarily produce more red blood cells than necessary. The production of more red blood cells results in thicker blood, which can lead to hemorrhage, thrombosis – the formation of blood clots inside blood vessels, and other medical complications. While there is no definitive cure for the condition, PV is primarily treated in two ways: phlebotomy and medication; these treatments can be offered individually or in conjunction with one another. Phlebotomies are performed on patients with PV – generally at regular intervals, such as weekly or monthly – to remove blood in an attempt to restore the patient's red blood cell count to normal. Additionally, certain medications may be administered to lower blood counts and/or to lower platelet counts in patients with PV.

HEMOPHILIA A

Hemophilia A is one of three hereditary coagulopathies; a coagulopathy is the term used to refer to any blood clotting disorder. The disorder affects approximately 70 to 90 percent of hemophiliacs. Hemophilia A is a blood clotting disorder characterized by the absence of blood clotting factor VIII. The inherited defective gene that causes hemophilia A is located on the X chromosome, which means that the condition primarily affects males, as males only have one X chromosome, and females have two; consequently, if a defect exists on a male's X chromosome, he does not have an additional X chromosome to compensate for the defect. Treatment is with cryoprecipitate.

VON WILLEBRAND DISEASE

Von Willebrand disease, one of three inherited coagulopathies, is characterized by an insufficient amount of von Willebrand factor in a patient's blood; von Willebrand factor assists with regular blood clotting, as it helps platelets join together and adhere to the walls of blood vessels. Symptoms of the disorder can include abnormally heavy menstrual bleeding in female patients; excessive nose bleeds; bruising – specifically, bruising that occurs in abnormal locations and/or unusually frequent bruising; and/or bleeding that occurs in a patient's mucous membranes, which can include the gums, the inside of the nose, and/or the lining of the intestinal tract. Prolonged bleeding from incisions or after surgery and skin irritations or rashes can be symptoms of von Willebrand disease as well.

MYELOFIBROSIS

Upon physical examination, a patient with myelofibrosis – a type of chronic leukemia in which scar tissue replaces bone marrow – will present with an enlarged spleen; if the condition has progressed to a certain stage, the physical examination may also reveal an enlarged liver. The progressive scarring of the bone marrow leads to the formation of blood in other areas of the body, such as the spleen and liver, which causes those organs to become enlarged in patients with the condition. When a complete blood count is obtained from a patient with myelofibrosis, the results will typically show variable platelet and white blood cell counts and a decreased red blood cell count. Additionally, upon observation, the red blood cells will appear to be shaped like teardrops.

ANEMIA

Anemia is a condition characterized by a deficiency of red blood cells in the blood. Red blood cells carry oxygen to tissue; consequently, a patient with anemia does not have an adequate oxygen supply to his/her tissue. Anemia can indicate potentially serious illnesses. Severe cases of the condition can lead to an inadequate supply of oxygen to the heart, which can ultimately lead to a heart attack. Without treatment, anemia can potentially cause a patient to develop a rapid or irregular heartbeat because the heart has to pump more blood to make up for the oxygen deficiency. Problems with the heart can additionally lead to congestive heart failure. Certain types of anemia can even cause nerve damage as well as a decrease in cognitive functioning due to the brain not receiving a sufficient amount of oxygen.

ASSESSING FOR HISTORY OF SICKLE CELL DISEASE PRIOR TO TRANSPORT

Situations that lead to hypoxia may cause problems for patients with sickle cell disease; consequently, patients should be assessed for the condition prior to transport. Flight transport can lead to hypoxia, a condition characterized by a deficit of oxygen within a patient's body, as the altitude of the transport vehicle increases and the oxygen pressure within the vehicle decreases.

Hypoxia can bring about sickling in patients with sickle cell disease, which causes capillary blood flow to become obstructed. Additionally, if the patient is being transported for a condition other than the sickle cell disease, the stress brought on by the reason for transport can also induce sickling. Accordingly, patients with the condition should always be transported with oxygen regardless of whether the condition is the primary reason for transport.

SICKLE CELL DISEASE

Sickle cell disease is a recessive genetic disorder of chromosome 11, causing hemoglobin to be defective so that red blood cells (RBCs) are sickle-shaped and inflexible, resulting in their accumulating in small vessels and causing painful blockage. While normal RBCs survive 120 days, sickled cells may survive only 10-20 days, stressing the bone marrow that can't produce fast enough and resulting in anemia. Different types of crises occur (aplastic, hemolytic, vaso-occlusive, and sequestrating), which cause infarctions in organs, severe pain, damage to organs, and rapid enlargement of liver and spleen. Sickle cell disease and crisis treatment includes:

- Intravenous fluids to prevent dehydration.
- Analgesics (morphine) during painful crises.
- Folic acid for anemia.
- Oxygen for congestive heart failure or pulmonary disease.
- Blood transfusions with chelation therapy to remove excess iron OR erythropheresis, in which red cells are removed and replaced with healthy cells, either autologous or from a donor.

Hematopoietic stem cells transplantation is the only curative treatment.

STANDARD PRECAUTIONS FOR INFECTION CONTROL

Standard precautions should be utilized for all patients because all body fluids (sweat, urine, feces, blood, sputum) and non-intact skin and mucous membranes may be infected:

Hand hygiene	Wash hands before and after each patient contact and after any contact with body fluids and contaminated items. Use soap and water for visible soiling.
Protective equipment	Use personal protective equipment (PPE), such as gloves, gowns, and masks, eye protection, and/or face shields, when anticipating contact with body fluids or contaminated skin.
Respiratory hygiene/ Cough etiquette	Utilize source control measures, such as covering cough, disposing of tissues, using surgical mask on person coughing or on staff to prevent inhalation of droplets, and properly disposing of dressings and used equipment. Wash hands after contacting respiratory secretions. Maintain a distance of >3 feet from coughing person when possible.

Soiled articles of clothing and linens should be handled as little as possible, and disposable items should be placed in leak-proof bags that can be burned.

TRANSMISSION-BASED PRECAUTIONS

The 2007 CDC isolation guidelines include both standard precautions that apply to all patients and transmission-based precautions for those with known or suspected infections as well as those with excessive wound drainage, other discharge, or fecal incontinence. Transmission-based precautions include:

Contact	Use personal protective equipment (PPE), including gown and gloves, for all contacts with the patient or patient's immediate environment.
Droplet	(Appropriate for influenza, streptococcus infection, pertussis, rhinovirus, and adenovirus and pathogens that remain viable and infectious for only short distances.) Use mask while caring for the patient. Maintain patient in > 3 feet away from other patients (with curtain separating in an emergency department. Use patient mask when transporting patient.
Airborne	(Appropriate for measles, chickenpox, tuberculosis, SARS because pathogens remain viable and infectious for long distances.) Use ≥N95 respirators (or masks) while caring for patient. Patient should be placed in an airborne infection isolation room in an emergency department.

TRANMISSION OF INFECTIOUS DISEASES THROUGH DROPLETS AND PARTICLES

When a person with an infectious disease coughs or sneezes, he/she sends droplets containing germs into the air. If a non-infected individual is within approximately three feet or less of the infected individual, the germ-carrying droplets can come in contact with the non-infected individual; the infectious disease germs are likely to cause symptoms of the illness in the non-infected individual if the droplets come in contact with that person's nose, mouth, or eyes. While particles are considerably smaller than droplets, their potential for transmitting infectious disease – such as tuberculosis – is quite large. Particles can carry germs that cause infectious diseases, and they can carry them through the air for extended periods of time; additionally, particles can travel in air currents. Consequently, if a non-infected individual inhales air that contains germs from an infectious disease, that individual will likely develop the disease.

MANAGING FEVER

A fever can accompany almost any kind of infection or illness. When a patient's core body temperature is at or above 100.4 degrees Fahrenheit (38 degrees Celsius), the patient is said to have a fever. Many times, a fever is simply the body's way of fighting an infection and may not pose a serious medical risk to the patient. However, a high fever may develop into further complications such as convulsions if left untreated. Certain medications including acetaminophen, aspirin, and ibuprofen are often effective at reducing a patient's fever. Additionally, the patient can be sponged with lukewarm water to assist in bringing his/her core body temperature back down to normal range. Patients with fevers should be encouraged to consume as much fluid as possible as well; clear fluids such as water and diluted juices are best.

SIRS AND SEPSIS

Systemic inflammatory response syndrome (SIRS), a generalized inflammatory response affecting may organ systems, may be caused by infectious or non-infectious agents, such as trauma, burns, adrenal insufficiency, pulmonary embolism, and drug overdose. If an infectious agent is identified or suspected, SIRS is an aspect of sepsis. SIRS includes 2 of the following:

- Elevated (>38°C) or subnormal rectal temperature (<36°C).
- Tachypnea (>20/min) or $PaCO_2$ <32 mmHg.
- Tachycardia >90/min.
- Leukocytosis (>12,000) or leukopenia (<4000) or >10% bands.

Sepsis is presence of infection either locally or systemically in which there is a generalized life-threatening inflammatory response (SIRS). It includes all the indications for SIRS as well as one of the following:

- Changes in mental status.
- Hypoxemia (<72 mmHg) without pulmonary disease.
- Elevation in plasma lactate.
- Systolic BP <90 mmHg or ≥40 mmHg below baseline.
- Decreased urinary output <5 mL/kg/wt for ≥1 hour.

If organs are affected, sepsis is classified as severe sepsis; and with hypotension, septic shock. MODS occurs with evidence of failure of 2 or more organs.

DENVER SEPSIS PROTOCOL

About a million cases of sepsis occur in the United States annually with incidence increasing, and about 25% of those with sepsis die, so rapidly identifying and treating sepsis is critical if the patient is to survive. The Denver Sepsis Protocol was developed to try to better respond to sepsis. The protocol is utilized if patients are 18, not pregnant, and have:

- SIRS: At least 2 criteria AND temperature >38° C (100.4° F) or <36° C (96° F), heart rate >90, respiration >20.
- Infection: Suspected/Documented.
- Hypotension or hypoperfusion with SBP <90, MAP <65, and lactate >4 mmol/L. (Utilizing portable lactate testing.)

PROTOCOL:
- Administer high flow oxygen with a non-rebreather mask.
- Insert two large-bore angiocaths and draw blood samples for baseline values.
- Administer IV fluid bolus at 20 mL/kg in rapid infusion.
- Reassess BP and respirations after infusion of 500 mL and contact physician if SBP <90 mmHg.
- Monitor vital signs (auscultate BP), ECG, pulse oximetry, capnography, glucose, and respirations regularly.

Patients should reach destination within 15 minutes and should receive antibiotics within one hour.

MANAGING PATIENTS WITH RISK OF HAVING A HIGHLY INFECTIOUS DISEASE

Patients diagnosed with or suspected of having highly infectious diseases, such as tuberculosis or meningitis, should be cared for utilizing the standard contact isolation procedures (gowns, gloves) as well as an airborne isolation procedures, which require the use of N95 respirators and eye protection during patient care. The patient should be transported to an airborne infection (negative pressure) isolation room in a receiving facility. Personal protective equipment (PPE) must be donned (beginning with mask, eye protection, gown, and gloves last) prior to patient contact. The patient should be masked before transport and air should be circulated continuously if possible. Disposable equipment should be used when possible as well as a closable emesis basins. The receiving facility should be made aware of the patient's infectious status. Any possible exposure should be reported immediately following protocols. In special circumstances, such as transport of Ebola patients, CDC guidelines for personal protection and isolation procedures must be followed exactly.

INTER-FACILITY TRANSFER AND POST TRANSPORT CLEANING ASSOCIATED WITH PATIENT WITH HIGHLY INFECTIOUS DISEASES

Before inter-facility transfer of a patient with a highly infectious disease, the CFRN should ensure that all necessary equipment is available in transport vehicles and that ground, flight and medical crewmembers are all aware of the patient's status and necessary isolation and decontamination procedures. Post-transport cleaning should correspond to CDC guidelines and should involve careful cleaning of all surfaces in proximity to the patient with removal of dust, body fluids, and debris before decontamination. The recommended decontamination agent for highly infectious agents is sodium hypochlorite (bleach) in a 1:100 dilution or pre-mixed wipes with one minute of contact needed to adequately kill organisms. Special cleaning supplies, such as Ambu-Stat®, an atomized cold sterilant solution, are also available. This type of fogger fills the vehicle with a sterilant and is used after surface cleaning. Critical and non-critical items should be cleaned and sterilized according to manufacturer's guidelines. Equipment left at the receiving facility must be properly cleaned or placed in a red bag before being returned to the transportation provider.

MEASURING CORE BODY TEMPERATURE

The hypothalamus is a mechanism in the brain responsible for controlling a person's core body temperature. The normal body temperature for a human is 98.6 degrees Fahrenheit (37.1 degrees Celsius). Core body temperature is most effectively measured by taking a patient's temperature rectally, which is the most common method of measuring temperature in a neonatal patient. However, if an adult patient is able to breathe through his/her nose without difficulty, temperature can also be measured orally by placing a thermometer underneath the patient's tongue. If an adult patient is not able to breathe through his/her nose due to illness or injury, temperature must be measured rectally, in an axillary position – in the patient's armpit, or in the ear. When taking a neonatal patient's temperature rectally, it is best to place the patient face down in order to carefully insert the thermometer a little over one centimeter into the anal canal.

HYPOTHERMIA

Hypothermia occurs when a person is not able to maintain a core body temperature at or above 95 degrees Fahrenheit (35 degrees Celsius). Subjective data to look at when determining whether a patient may be suffering from the condition can include: the geographic location of the patient and the corresponding temperature of the surroundings in which he/she is located; how appropriately the patient is dressed in relation to the temperature of his/her surroundings; the length of time the patient was exposed to conditions that may contribute to the development of hypothermia; and whether or not the patient has medical risk factors for developing the condition. Risk factors for hypothermia can include: 1) patient age – older and very young patients may be more susceptible to hypothermia; 2) certain medical conditions such as Parkinson's disease and stroke; and 3) mental impairment such as Alzheimer's disease and alcohol or drug use.

Mild, moderate, and severe hypothermia are described below:

- Mild hypothermia: occurs when a patient has a core body temperature less than 95 degrees Fahrenheit (35 degrees Celsius) and greater than 89.6 degrees Fahrenheit (32 degrees Celsius); patients with mild hypothermia have a very low risk of dying from the condition.
- Moderate hypothermia: occurs when a patient has a core body temperature less than 89.6 degrees Fahrenheit (32 degrees Celsius) and greater than 82.4 degrees Fahrenheit (28 degrees Celsius).

- Severe hypothermia: occurs when a patient has a core body temperature at or below 82.4 degrees Fahrenheit (28 degrees Celsius); patients with severe hypothermia are at an increased risk of dying from the condition than those with mild or moderate forms of hypothermia.

RESTORING CORE BODY TEMPERATURE

In patients whose core body temperature is too high or too low, it is important to monitor the patient's airway, breathing, and circulation periodically during transport. To help restore a patient's core body temperature when it has dropped too low, the patient can be wrapped in insulated blankets during transport. Warm gel packs can also be applied to areas of the body to help elevate the core body temperature. If the patient has any articles of clothing on his/her body that appear to be wet, it is best to remove those articles to prevent a further decrease in temperature. If available, warm fluids can be administered to the patient as well.

SYMPTOMS OF FROSTBITE

Upon physical examination, a patient with frostbite may present with pale or bluish colored skin. A patient with bluish colored skin may be displaying signs of not having enough oxygen in his/her blood. Necrosis may occur when not enough blood is being pumped to the area(s) where the frostbite is located. Necrosis occurs when portions of tissue or portions of an organ stop functioning; bluish or purplish regions on the body may indicate this condition. Edema – swelling of an organ or tissue as a result of a build-up of lymph fluid – may also be present in patients with frostbite. At the area(s) where the frostbite is located, the patient may not be as sensitive to touch, due to decreased sensation in and around those areas.

Treatment for frostbite includes rapid rewarming with a warm water bath (40–42°C, 104–107.6°F) for 10–30 minutes or until the frostbitten area is erythematous and pliable as well as treatment for generalized hypothermia. After warming, treatment includes debridement of clear blisters but not hemorrhagic blisters. Frostbite most often affects the nose, ears, and distal extremities. As frostbite develops, the affected part feels numb and aches or throbs, becoming hard and insensate as the tissue freezes, resulting in circulatory impairment, necrosis of tissue, and gangrene. Three zones of injury include:

- Coagulation (usually distal): severe irreversible cellular damage
- Hyperemia (usually proximal): minimal cellular damage
- Stasis (between other two zones): severe but sometimes reversible damage

CARDIAC ARRHYTHMIA AS CAUSE OF DEATH IN HYPOTHERMIA VICTIMS

During early stages of hypothermia, when the condition would be classified as mild, patients almost always experience an increase in heart rate for a brief period of time. As the core body temperature of the patient decreases, as it does when hypothermia progresses from mild to moderate to severe stages, the patient's heart rate also begins to decrease. At core body temperatures lower than 91.4 degrees Fahrenheit (33 degrees Celsius), the heart can decrease to a rate of 20 beats per minute. When a patient's heart rate fluctuates as it commonly does when hypothermia sets in, the fluctuation can lead to cardiac arrhythmia, which is a condition characterized by an irregular or abnormal heart rate.

RESTORING HEAT STROKE PATIENT'S CORE BODY TEMPERATURE

In patients whose core body temperature is too high or too low, it is important to monitor the patient's airway, breathing, and circulation periodically during transport. To help restore a patient's core body temperature when it is too high, it is often helpful to dampen the patient's skin with cool water using a misting technique. If a cooling blanket is available during the transport process, place the patient on the device. Additionally, cold packs may be applied to the patient's neck, groin area, and/or under the arms. Administer fluids to the patient in a manner that prevents fluid overload, which could lead to pulmonary edema. The patient's urine production should be closely monitored during transport, as it is necessary for heat stroke patients to produce more urine than usual to avoid the risk of developing acute renal failure.

DECOMPRESSION SICKNESS

Decompression sickness occurs when a patient is exposed to an abrupt decrease in either the water or air pressure around him/her. The condition can be characterized by symptoms including limb pain, decreased respiratory functioning, skin reactions, and it can lead to problems related to the central nervous system such as headaches, confusion, and diminished motor skills. Patients should be treated at a hyperbaric compression chamber. Due to the nature of the disorder, if a patient with decompression sickness must be transported via flight, the trip should be flown at an altitude no higher than 3000 feet. To prevent circulatory collapse, the patient must be transported to the chamber within a period of six hours or less from the onset of the condition. During transport, the patient should be administered 100 percent oxygen to relieve the deprivation of oxygen to the tissues, a condition known as tissue hypoxia.

ENVENOMATION

Envenomation can occur from a variety of animal bites including certain types of fish such as jellyfish and stingrays, poisonous snakes such as pit vipers, and spiders such as Black Widows. Common signs of envenomation in a patient include swelling at the site of venom injection, redness and pain at the site, gastrointestinal problems, and neurological issues. Gastrointestinal-related symptoms may include diarrhea and/or nausea/vomiting as well as abdominal discomfort or pain. Neurological symptoms may include dizziness, numbness at the injection site, and lethargy. Envenomation may also cause hypotension and bradycardia.

CARING FOR PATIENT ENVENOMATED BY POISONOUS SNAKE

Once it has been determined that the patient has been envenomated, the injured body part should be immobilized, which can help limit the amount of venom that circulates throughout the patient's bloodstream. In all envenomation cases, the flight team should make every effort to help the patient remain calm, which also helps decrease venom circulation throughout the bloodstream. Additionally, the patient's airway, breathing, and overall circulation should be consistently and closely monitored during transport to ensure that the reaction to the snake bite remains local and not systemic. A large-bore IV line should be established in the patient – away from the location of the bite, if possible. Analgesia can be given to the patient for pain. Treatment is largely dependent on the type of envenomation sustained. Severe local pain and edema (signs of mild envenomation) around the bite site are indications for antivenin (5 vials). Because some bites are "dry" and antivenin is expensive, not readily available, and can have significant side effects, it is not given on request or without evidence of envenomation. Fang marks and some pain and local tenderness are common from trauma without envenomation. Moderate envenomation may include swelling beyond the area of bite, mild coagulopathy, and systemic manifestation with increasing symptoms with severe or life-threatening envenomation. Treatment may include 5–25 vials of antivenin, depending on the grade of envenomation and symptoms.

EXPOSURE TO TOXIC SUBSTANCES

When a patient intentionally exposes him/herself to a toxic substance or substances, the result is known as an overdose. Patients can also be exposed to toxic substances inadvertently. Unintentional exposure to toxic substances is usually caused by medication errors, food poisoning, environmental sources, and/or bites or stings from animals or insects that transfer toxins into the patient's bloodstream. Medication errors occur when a patient or caregiver incorrectly reads a label and ingests too much of a particular medication. Pediatric patients are often victims of unintentional exposure to toxic substances, as medication bottles often pique their curiosity, and, subsequently, cause medical complications if they ingest the medication.

N-acetylcysteine is the antidote for acetaminophen toxicity and is most effective in protecting the liver if given within 8 hours. Toxicity is plotted on the Rumack–Matthew nomogram with serum levels of more than 150 mg requiring an antidote. The 72-hour N-acetylcysteine protocol includes 140 mg/kg initially and 70 mg/kg every 4 hours for seventeen more doses.

Hydroxocobalamin is the preferred treatment of choice for cyanide toxicity with the dose of 70 mg/kg IV. Nitrites (found in some cyanide treatment kits) displace oxygen on the hemoglobin molecules, forming methemoglobin, thereby reducing the ability of hemoglobin to carry sufficient oxygen, and may result in unstable hemodynamic status.

MEDICAL MANAGEMENT FOR INGESTED TOXIC SUBSTANCE

The first component of managing of a patient who has ingested a toxic substance is to evaluate his/her airway, breathing, and circulation. The patient's heart and lungs should also be evaluated to ensure that the cardiopulmonary system is functioning properly. It is important to manage the symptoms of the toxic substance ingestion as well as managing the toxic substance itself by attempting to prevent the substance from being absorbed into the stomach. Absorption can potentially be prevented by using activated charcoal, by performing whole bowel irrigation, or through nasogastric aspiration. Activated charcoal effectively absorbs most toxic substances. For substances that are not absorbed by charcoal, flushing out the gastrointestinal tract through whole bowel irrigation may be necessary. Placing a tube down a patient's nose into his/her stomach and suctioning out the contents – a procedure known as nasogastric aspiration – may also be necessary for substances that cannot be absorbed by charcoal.

DRUG OVERDOSE

Given the vast number of drugs available, symptoms of drug overdose vary widely and depend on the specific drug. The pupils of a drug overdose patient may not appear normal; they may appear enlarged/dilated or extremely small like pin points, or they may also appear unchanging and stay their normal size when exposed to light. Sweating, shakiness, and convulsions can also be symptoms of a drug overdose. A patient's behavior can provide further indications of a possible drug overdose. Patients who overdose often act delusional or paranoid, and they tend to become agitated and aggressive relatively easily. They may also have hallucinations as a result of the substance abuse. Patients who act unusually drowsy and/or who have an unstable gait may be exhibiting symptoms of an overdose as well. Breathing difficulties such as rapid breathing, shallow breathing, or labored breathing can also be indications of a drug overdose.

DELIRIUM TREMENS

Chronic abuse of ethanol (alcoholism) is associated with alcohol withdrawal syndrome *(delirium tremens)* with abrupt cessation of alcohol intake, resulting in hallucinations, tachycardia, diaphoresis, and sometimes-psychotic behavior. It may be precipitated by trauma or infection and has a high mortality rate, 5-15% with treatment and 35% without treatment. Management includes:

- Monitor vital signs and blood gases.
- Use the Clinical Instrument for Withdrawal for Alcohol (CIWA) to measure symptoms of withdrawal.
- Assess and monitor level of consciousness, orientation, alterations in sensory impressions, agitation, and anxiety.
- Provide an environment with minimal sensory stimulus (lower lights, close blinds).
- Implement fall and seizure precautions.
- Provide nutritional support and monitor intake and output.
- Implement measures to assure proper sleep and stress management.
- Express acceptance and reassurance.
- Maintain body temperature.

People easily aroused can usually safely sleep off the effects of ingesting too much alcohol but if semi-conscious or unconscious, emergency medical treatment (such as IV fluids and medications, intubation, and/or dialysis) may be necessary.

MILD TO MODERATE SYMPTOMS OF SUBSTANCE USE WITHDRAWAL

Patients who experience symptoms of withdrawal when they stop using alcohol or other substances often experience both physical and psychological symptoms. Similar to drug overdose symptoms, symptoms of withdrawal vary widely depending on the patient and depending on the substance in question. Mild to moderate physical symptoms of withdrawal can include headaches, nausea and/or vomiting, appetite loss, clammy and/or pale skin, heart palpitations, abnormal pupil size, difficulty sleeping, and sweating. While they may have a difficult time actually sleeping, fatigue is another common symptom of withdrawal. Psychological withdrawal symptoms that would be considered mild or moderate may include feelings of anxiety, depression, excitability, nervousness, irritability, and swift changes from one emotion to another. Additionally, patients going through withdrawal often have a difficult time thinking clearly.

TREATMENT FOR TOXIC INGESTIONS

Treatment for toxic ingestions is related to the type of toxin and whether or not it is identified:

- Administration of reversal agent if substance is known and an antidote exists. Antidotes for common toxins include:
  - Opiates: Naloxone (Narcan®)
  - Toxic alcohols: Ethanol infusion and/or dialysis
  - Acetaminophen: N-acetylcysteine
  - Calcium channel blockers, beta-blockers: Calcium chloride, Glucagon
  - Tricyclic antidepressants: Sodium bicarbonate
  - Ethylene glycol: fomepizole
  - Iron: deferoxamine
- GI decontamination at one time was standard procedures (Ipecac® and gastric lavage followed by activated charcoal). It is no longer advised for routine use although selective gastric lavage may be appropriate if done within 1 hour of ingestion
- Activated charcoal (1 g/kg/wt) orally or per NG tube binds to many toxins if given within one hour of ingestion. It may also be used in multiple doses (q 4-6 hrs) to enhance elimination

Forced diuresis with alkalinization of urine (>7.5) may prevent absorption of drugs that are weak bases or acids.

ACTIVATED CHARCOAL

Activated charcoal is often administered to a patient who has ingested a toxic substance or overdosed on a drug. It is intended to absorb the substance or drug and safely eliminate it from the patient's body before it reaches the stomach. While activated charcoal can be effective against certain forms of poisoning, it is ineffective at absorbing others; therefore, its use is not advisable when such poisons are involved. The use of activated charcoal is not advised when a patient has ingested acids, alkalis, iron, lithium, alcohols, and/or products containing petroleum such as cleaning agents, coal or fuel oil, and paint thinner. Gastrointestinal decontamination is most effective if done within 1 hour of ingestion, although activated charcoal may have some protective effects if given within 4 hours of ingestion.

DISTRIBUTIVE SHOCK

Distributive shock occurs with adequate blood volume but inadequate intravascular volume because of arterial/venous dilation that results in decreased vascular tone and hypoperfusion of internal organs. Cardiac output may be normal or blood may pool, decreasing cardiac output. Distributive shock may result from anaphylactic shock, septic shock, neurogenic shock, and drug ingestions.

Symptoms	Treatment
Hypotension (systolic <90mm Hg or <40mm Hg from nor-mal), tachypnea, tachycardia (>90) (may be lower if patient receiving β-blockers. Skin initially warm, later hypoperfused. Hyper- or hypothermia (>38°C or <36°C). Hypoxemia. Alterations in mentation. Decreased Urinary output. Symptoms related to underlying cause.	Treating underlying cause and stabilizing hemodynamics: Septic shock or anaphylactic therapy and monitoring as indicated. Oxygen with endotracheal intubation if necessary. Rapid fluid administration at 0.25-0.5L NS or isotonic crystalloid every 5-10 minutes as needed to 2-3 L. Inotropic agents (dopamine, dobutamine, norepinephrine) if necessary.

MANAGEMENT OF PATIENT WITH OBSTRUCTIVE SHOCK

Obstructive shock occurs when venous return to the heart (preload) is impeded because of some type of obstruction or direct compression of the heart. Common causes include:

- Pulmonary embolism: Hypotension (SBP <90 mmHg), tachypnea, tachycardia, and cough. Treatment is anticoagulation or thrombolysis.
- Pneumothorax (often associated with fractured rib): Onset is rapid with pallor, hypotension, tachycardia, impaired peripheral circulation, tachypnea, and chest pain decreased or absent breath sounds on affected side. Tracheal deviation is a late indication. Treatment is needle thoracostomy (14 gauge, 3.25 inch) followed by chest tube insertion.
- Pericardial tamponade: Beck's triad (hypotension, muffled heart sounds, and JVD), ECG changes (slow or varying QRS), or tachycardia. Percutaneous drainage under ultrasound guidance may relieve severe symptoms, but patient may require immediate surgical intervention.

In all cases, provide oxygen to maintain oxygen saturation of at least 94%, start an IV line, monitor ECG, keep warm, lie flat or in position of comfort, and transport rapidly.

ANAPHYLAXIS

Anaphylaxis syndrome may present with a few symptoms or a wide range that encompasses cardiopulmonary, dermatological, and gastrointestinal responses.

Symptoms	Treatments
Symptoms may recur after the initial treatment (biphasic anaphylaxis), so careful monitoring is essential: Sudden onset of weakness, dizziness, confusion. Severe generalized edema and angioedema. Lips and tongue may swell. Urticaria Increased permeability of vascular system and loss of vascular tone. Severe hypotension leading to shock. Laryngospasm/bronchospasm with obstruction of airway causing dyspnea and wheezing. Nausea, vomiting, and diarrhea. Seizures, coma and death.	Establish patent airway and intubate if necessary for ventilation. Provide oxygen at 100% high flow. Monitor VS. Administer epinephrine (Epi-pen® or solution). Albuterol per nebulizer for bronchospasm. Intravenous fluids to provide bolus of fluids for hypotension. Diphenhydramine if shock persists. Methylprednisolone if no response to other drugs.

HYPOVOLEMIC SHOCK

Hypovolemic shock occurs when the total circulating volume of fluid decreases, leading to a fall in venous return that in turn causes a decrease in ventricular filling and preload, indicated by ↓ in right atrial pressure (RAP) and pulmonary artery occlusion pressure (PAOP). This results in a decrease in stroke volume and cardiac output. This in turn causes generalized arterial vasoconstriction, increasing afterload (↑ systemic vascular resistance), causing decreased tissue perfusion.

Symptoms	Treatment
Anxiety. Pallor. Cool and clammy skin. Delayed capillary refill Cyanosis. Hypotension. Increasing respirations. Weak, thready pulse.	Treatment is aimed at identifying and treating the cause of fluid loss and reestablishing an adequate intravascular volume of fluid through administration of blood, blood products, autotransfusion, colloids (such as plasma protein fraction), and/or crystalloids (such as normal saline). Oxygen may be given and intubation and ventilation may be necessary. Medications may include vasopressors, such as dopamine.

Trauma

PRIMARY ASSESSMENT OF TRAUMA PATIENT

During the primary assessment of a trauma patient – which should be performed rapidly – the airway and cervical spine should be stabilized first. Following stabilization of the airway and cervical spine, the patient's breathing and ventilation should be assessed. Upon assessing breathing and ventilation, circulation should be evaluated, and any active hemorrhaging should be controlled with direct pressure. Fourth, the patient's neurological state should be assessed to determine any decrease in cognitive functioning. Finally, the patient should be undressed in order to identify and treat any previously missed trauma sites and/or injuries.

SECONDARY ASSESSMENT OF TRAUMA PATIENT

The secondary assessment of a trauma patient involves an extensive visual scan of the patient to identify all sustained injuries; consequently, it is most beneficial for the patient to be completely undressed prior to this scan. If it is not feasible for the patient to be fully disrobed, the patient's chest and abdomen should at least be exposed. Restrictive attire such as belts should be removed or cut off. To prevent cold-related emergencies in trauma patients, areas of the patient's body that are not being examined should be covered with blankets. The purpose of the secondary assessment is to reveal injuries; the flight team does not treat specific injuries during this process. To avoid losing valuable time that could be spent treating injuries, it is imperative that the secondary assessment be performed in a quick manner. Inspection, auscultation, palpation, and history taking are essential components of the secondary assessment.

TRAUMA SCORE

The Trauma Score is an index that rates physiological characteristics of patients. These characteristics include: 1) systolic blood pressure; 2) respiratory rate; 3) respiratory expansion; 4) capillary refill; and 5) score on the Glasgow Coma Scale. The original Trauma Scale has been revised to include characteristics one, two, and five described above – systolic blood pressure, respiratory rate, and Glasgow Coma Scale score. The Glasgow Coma Scale rates patients in terms of eye response, verbal response, and motor response. Patients are given a score between three and 15, where a score of three to eight indicates severe brain injury, nine to 12 indicates moderate brain injury, and 13 to 15 indicates mild injury. The three parameters of the Revised Trauma Score combined offer a means of predicting patient survival. A higher Revised Trauma Score correlates with a higher probability of survival.

INJURIES LIKELY TO RESULT FROM MOTOR VEHICLE CRASHES

If a driver is not wearing a safety restraint during a motor vehicle crash, head and facial injuries are likely to occur. Additionally, the larynx, sternum, patella, femur, and clavicle are structures that often fracture during a crash when a driver is unrestrained. Cardiac contusion and organ or blood vessel laceration also occur frequently in crashes involving unrestrained drivers. If a driver is wearing a safety restraint when a motor vehicle crash occurs, he/she will likely sustain injuries either from the lap restraint or from the shoulder restraint. Injuries that are often caused by a lap restraint include injuries to the pelvis, spleen, liver, and/or pancreas. Injuries frequently sustained from a shoulder restraint include cervical fractures and injuries to the mitral valve or diaphragm. The mitral valve and diaphragm often rupture as a result of injury sustained from a shoulder restraint during a motor vehicle crash.

ARTERIAL AND VENOUS INJURIES

Arterial injuries are characterized by abundant hemorrhaging from open wounds. Venous injuries also have the capacity to produce hemorrhaging from open or closed wounds; however, bleeding from venous injuries is not as plentiful as it is with arterial injuries. Edema – swelling of an organ or tissue as a result of a build-up of lymph fluid – is present in venous injuries. The temperature of the injured area can also help differentiate an arterial injury from a venous one. The site of an arterial injury will be cool in temperature while a venous injury site may either be cool or warm. It is common to see poor capillary filling associated with arterial injuries; capillary filling tends to be good following a venous injury. Both types of injuries may be accompanied by a diminished pulse, but a patient with an arterial injury may also lack a pulse altogether.

SELECTION OF WOUND DRESSING

The location of the wound – whether it is located superficially or whether it has become a full thickness or cavity wound – should be considered prior to selecting a dressing. Next, a description of the wound should be determined. A necrotic wound is comprised of dead tissue and is often characterized by a black, leathery appearance. A sloughy wound is one characterized by a thick yellow layer covering the wound, while a granulating wound may be characterized by a bright red color; a granulating wound may appear to be shiny, and it may bleed easily. Characteristics of the wound including factors such as whether it is dry or moist and whether it is painful should also be taken into consideration before dressing a wound. The wound's bacterial profile – whether it is sterile, infected, or infected with the potential to cross-infect – is also an important attribute to consider when selecting a dressing.

CONTROLLING VISIBLE HEMORRHAGE

Many types of hemorrhage exist, but hemorrhage in the general sense means severe bleeding or significant loss of blood. When the source of a patient's blood loss can be visualized, there are ways to control the hemorrhage. First and foremost, the patient's airway, breathing, and circulation should be assessed. Once those have been evaluated, the hemorrhage site should be freed from constrictive clothing or attire of any kind so that the site is exposed. In cases of minor bleeding, direct pressure should be applied to the injury site to stop the bleeding, the site should be cleansed with soap and water, and a sterile dressing should be applied. In cases of serious hemorrhage, the risks of causing further damage to an injured site should be considered against the possible benefits of applying direct pressure to the area.

TOURNIQUETS

Tourniquets are recommended as life-saving devices for uncontrolled arterial hemorrhage of the extremities that cannot be controlled with pressure or other means. The types of trauma tourniquets that are recommended were developed by the military but are now in common use for emergency care. The Combat Application Tourniquet ® (CAT) and the SOF Tactical Tourniquet® (SOF-T) are adjustable bands with a windlass stick to tighten and a windlass clip and strap. The tourniquet is applied about 2 inches above the wound or above the knee for lower leg wounds and above the elbow for lower arm wounds. After the tourniquet is applied, the windlass is twisted to tighten until the distal pulse disappears and bleeding slows considerably or stops. Once bleeding is controlled, the windlass is secured. The tourniquet should be kept open to the field of vision so it is constantly monitored. If no tourniquet is available, a BP cuff can be applied and inflated.

EMERGENCY PELVIC STABILIZATION

Patients with pelvic fractures are at risk for significant blood loss and hypovolemia. Pelvic fractures should be suspected with high impact injuries, such as falls from a high place or pedestrian-motor vehicle accidents. Patients may complain of abdominal or back pain, pain in the pelvic area, and/or numbness and tingling of the lower extremities. Excessive palpation or manipulation should be avoided and the pelvis should be stabilized with a circumferential pressure device (remove items from pockets first):

- Sheet wrap: A draw sheet is folded horizontally and made about 1 foot wide, placed beneath the patient, wrapped tightly around the pelvic area, and secured with clamps or other means.
- T-POD: Slide the belt under patient and around patient, adjust size to leave a 6 inch space between belt ends. Attach the velcro pulley system to each side of belt, then adjust pull-tabs to increase circumferential pressure. Finally, secure compression.
- SAM pelvic sling: Place belt under hips and wrap around. Fasten belt snugly, and secure.

TRACTION SPLINTS

Traction splints are applied to mid-shaft fractures of the femur (if no other leg fracture, severe injury, or pelvic fractures are present) to stabilize bone ends, reduce bleeding and relieve discomfort. At least 2 people are usually needed when applying the traction splint and constant communication is necessary. Procedure:

- Stabilize leg and apply gentle steady manual traction.
- Check motor function (move toes), sensation, and distal pulse.
- Apply ankle hitch.
- Position traction device (the Hare® device is placed under the leg and the Sagar® to the medial aspect of the leg) and secure proximal and then distal straps.
- Attach ankle hitch to the device.
- Apply traction slowly (maximum 10% of body weight or 15 pounds for Sagar®), using the uninjured leg as a guide to length if leg distorted.
- Reassess distal circulation.
- Place patient on backboard and secure traction device to the backboard.

If incorrectly applied, the traction splint can increased bleeding, damage nerves and soft tissue, and increase the risk of compartment syndrome.

RAPID VOLUME RESUSCITATION

Rapid volume resuscitation in a shock patient can be accompanied by serious medical complications for the patient if it is not performed correctly. The amount of fluid a shock patient needs varies from patient to patient; it is dependent upon the volume of fluid loss that has occurred within the blood vessels. During resuscitation efforts, it is particularly important that transport team members carefully monitor the patient's blood pressure, pulse, urinary output, and awareness level. Parameters such as these can indicate when a patient has received a sufficient level of volume resuscitation, and they can also indicate when a patient has received too much fluid during resuscitation efforts. The transport team should also constantly monitor the shock patient for signs of complications resulting from the rapid volume resuscitation.

INDICATIONS FOR INFUSION OF FRESH FROZEN PLASMA AND INFUSION OF PLATELETS

Fresh frozen plasma may be infused to correct hemorrhage or an anticipated large volume blood loss. It can also be used to increase a patient's clotting factor if the patient is deficient. An infused unit of fresh frozen plasma can increase a patient's clotting factor by two to three percent if he/she is average size. Additionally, platelets may be infused in an attempt to increase a patient's clotting factor. They can also be infused to overcome bleeding in a patient with thrombocytopenia, which is a condition characterized by a low platelet count. An infused unit of platelets can increase a patient's platelet count by 5,000 or more if he/she is average size. Patients experiencing hemorrhage, septic shock, or coagulation defects may warrant platelet infusions.

Safe Administration of Blood Products

Emergency blood product transfusions are usually of plasma and packed red blood cells (PRBCs). Before administration, the CFRN should check the dates and temperature of the blood supply (generally in a transport cooler). If the blood type was specifically supplied for a patient, the blood type and name should be verified; but for emergency purposes, type O is generally all that is available, as it can be administered to most people without reaction. Indications include hemodynamic instability and acute hypoperfusion with systolic BP <90 and pulse rate >120 from hemorrhage (traumatic or internal), penetrating chest wound, ruptured aortic aneurysm, or patient-specific hemoglobin (such as less than 7 mg/dL) with ongoing bleeding (such as from GI hemorrhage). Protocols may vary, but generally one unit of plasma and one unit of PRBCs are administered through warmed infusions (to patients 12 or older) and orders sought for additional units. Vital signs, temperature, and patient assessment should be monitored throughout the transfusion, and the receiving facility must be notified of the transfusion.

Outline Recommended Blood Pressure Levels

Blood pressure can range from low to normal to prehypertension to high. Normal blood pressure is characterized by a systolic pressure of less than 120 millimeters of mercury (mmHg) and a diastolic pressure of less than 80 mmHg. Patients whose systolic pressure falls within the range of 120 to 139 mmHg or whose diastolic pressure falls within the range of 80 to 89 mmHg are categorized as having prehypertension. High blood pressure can be categorized as stage 1 or stage 2, with stage 2 being more dangerous. Stage 1 high blood pressure is characterized by a systolic pressure of 140 to 159 mmHg or a diastolic pressure of 90 to 99 mmHg; stage 2 is defined as a systolic pressure of 160 mmHg or above or a diastolic pressure 100 mmHg or greater.

Cardiogenic Shock

Cardiogenic shock in adults most often is secondary to myocardial infarction damage that reduces the contractibility of the ventricles, interfering with the pumping mechanism of the heart, decreasing oxygen perfusion. Cardiogenic shock has 3 characteristics: Increased preload, increased afterload, and decreased contractibility. Together these result in a decreased cardiac output and an increase in systemic vascular resistance (SVR) to compensate and protect vital organs. This results in an increase of afterload in the left ventricle with increased need for oxygen. As the cardiac output continues to decrease, tissue perfusion decreases, coronary artery perfusion decreases, fluid backs up and the left ventricle fails to adequately pump the blood, resulting in pulmonary edema and right ventricular failure. Decreasing oxygen consumption is a major initial goal of cardiogenic shock.

Symptoms	Treatment
Hypotension with systolic BP <90 mm Hg	IV fluids
Tachycardia > 100 beats/min with weak thready pulse and dysrhythmias	Inotropic agents
	Antidysrhythmics
Decreased heart sounds	IABP or left ventricular assist device
Chest pain	
Tachypnea and basilar rales	
Cool, moist skin, pallor	

INTRAOSSEOUS NEEDLE PLACEMENT

Once the need for inserting an intraosseous needle has been determined, the following steps should be taken during the placement of the needle:

- Wearing a mask and sterile gloves, the insertion site should be cleansed.
- Identify and palpate the tibia, the larger of the two leg bones located below the knee.
- Insert the needle in the skin that covers the flat surface of the tibia.
- With the needle at approximately a 10 to 30-degree angle, advance the needle through the periosteum of the tibia, the tissue that covers the bone.
- Continue advancing the needle into the bone using a twisting motion.
- When the needle is in the marrow cavity of the tibia – the correct location for the needle – a decreased level of resistance will be felt.
- After removing the stylet from the needle, attach intravenous tubing, and secure the needle.

SELDINGER TECHNIQUE FOR INSERTING A CVC

Following the Seldinger technique for central venous catheter (CVC) insertion, a sharp, hollow needle is used to puncture a blood vessel. Once the needle has punctured the site, a guidewire is advanced through the needle's cavity, and the needle is withdrawn from the site. A flexible tube – or cannula – that can be used either to remove fluid or to administer medication is then passed over the guidewire, and the guidewire is withdrawn. The cannula can also be used to position a catheter, if necessary. Once the fluid has been withdrawn and/or the medication has been delivered to the patient through the CVC, the cannula is removed, and the procedure is complete.

SHOCK

There are a number of different types of shock, but there are general characteristics that they have in common. In all types of shock, there is a marked decrease in tissue perfusion related to hypotension, so that there is insufficient oxygen delivered to the tissues and, in turn, inadequate removal of cellular waste products, causing injury to tissue:

- Hypotension (systolic below 90 mm Hg). This may be somewhat higher (110 mm Hg) in those who are initially hypertensive.
- Decreased urinary output (<0.5 mL/kg/hr), especially marked in hypovolemic shock
- Metabolic acidosis.
- Hypoxemia <90 mm Hg for children and adults birth-50; < 80mm Hg for those 51 to 70 and <70 for those over 70.
- Peripheral/cutaneous vasoconstriction/vasodilation resulting in cool, clammy skin.
- Alterations in level of consciousness.

	Distributive	Cardiogenic	Hypovolemic
Preload	↓ (sometimes stays same)	↑	↓
Cardiac Output	↑	↓	↓
SVR	↓	↑	↑

CARDIOVASCULAR TRAUMA

The following are four types of cardiovascular trauma:

- Myocardial contusion – bruising of the heart muscle typically caused by trauma such as a long-distance fall, a crushing motor vehicle accident, or too much pressure applied during cardiopulmonary resuscitation attempts; this type of cardiovascular trauma can lead to the heart moving in an abnormal manner
- Aortic dissection – tear occurring in the aorta, which is the main artery leaving the heart; when a patient experiences an aortic dissection, blood can flow in directions it does not typically flow and/or can pool in certain areas and lead to aneurysm; blunt-force traumas such as crushing motor vehicle accidents are often the cause of aortic dissections
- Pericardial tamponade – build-up of fluid in the membranes surrounding the heart, known as the pericardium; medical conditions are the typical causes of this type of cardiovascular trauma, but blunt-force trauma to the chest can also result in pericardial tamponade
- Vascular injury – any injury caused by trauma to the blood vessels, muscle, or tissues

MYOCARDIAL CONTUSION, PULMONARY CONTUSION, AND RIB FRACTURE

A myocardial contusion occurs when the heart muscle is bruised. Patients often sustain myocardial contusion from motor vehicle accidents, aggressive chest compressions during cardiopulmonary resuscitation (CPR) efforts, and/or blunt chest trauma resulting from a fall. Symptoms of the condition are typically mild. Many patients with myocardial contusion feel as though their heart is racing, and they also frequently experience pain in their breastbone. A pulmonary contusion occurs when the lung becomes bruised. High-velocity motor vehicle accidents are a common cause of pulmonary contusion. Symptoms of the condition may include the presence of rales during inhalation, an increased rate of respiration, and/or breathing difficulties. Rib fractures most often occur as a result of trauma to the chest. Similar to myocardial and pulmonary contusions, symptoms of broken ribs tend to be somewhat mild. Patients with rib fractures generally experience pain when the fracture site is pressed upon and pain upon deep inhalation.

TUBE THORACOSTOMY

A tube thoracostomy is the procedure by which a tube is inserted in a patient's chest. The purpose of the chest tube is to remove fluid or air that has entered the pleural space – located between the inner and outer linings of the lung – as it can cause the patient's lung to collapse. If the fluid and/or air can be removed through the chest tube, the lungs will be able to expand completely, and the risk of collapse will be minimized. Pneumothorax – air accumulation in the pleural space – and pleural effusion – fluid accumulation in the pleural space – are two primary conditions for which a tube thoracostomy is indicated. The procedure is generally indicated for any condition or situation that could lead to a collapsed lung such as hemothorax, which is characterized by bleeding into the chest; empyema, an accumulation of pus in the pleural space; chest trauma; or chest surgery.

A tube thoracostomy is the procedure whereby a tube is inserted into a patient's chest in an attempt to remove fluid or air. Prior to the procedure, if the patient can tolerate it, provide pain control and local anesthesia ans well as supplemental oxygen. Once the area has been anesthetized, prep skin with chlorhexidine and perform procedure using sterile procedure and full barrier precautions. Make a small incision parallel to the intercostal space. Then use a Kelly clamp to dissect and make a little tunnel through which the tube will be inserted. Clamp the chest tube with the Kelly clamp and then insert the chest tube into the tunnel that was created. After placing, remove the clamp and look for condensation in the tube on respiration or any drainage, making sure all drainage holes are within the thoracic space. To prevent the tube from falling out, it is sutured to or taped to the patient's skin. Obtain x-rays when able. Monitor lung expansion, breath sounds, oxygenation status and vitals.

ASSESSING CHEST TUBE AND DRAINAGE SYSTEM

After the chest tube and drainage system have been inserted, the patient's level of comfort should be evaluated and, if possible, adjustments should be made to achieve an optimal comfort level. While the tube is in place, breath sounds and breathing rate should be monitored for abnormalities or changes that occur. Additionally, the patient's heart rate, blood pressure, and core body temperature should be monitored continuously. Oxygen saturation levels should be obtained to ensure that they are within normal range. The amount, color, and consistency of any drainage should be documented periodically while the drainage system is in place and assess and document bubbling in the water seal or whether the chest tube is to suction and if so how much suction. Subcutaneous emphysema, a condition whereby the skin covering the chest wall allows air to penetrate the patient's tissues, can occur at the site where the chest tube was inserted; consequently, the flight team member should assess for the condition by palpating the chest wall and listening for a crackling sensation. Tubing should be kept from kinking.

ACS SYMPTOMS

Abdominal compartment syndrome (ACS) occurs when intraabdominal pressure (IAP) is sustained at >20 mmHg (normal 0-5 mmHg), resulting in multi-organ failure and death. ACS may be primary, caused by abdominal trauma, ruptured aortic aneurysm, or retroperitoneal hemorrhage associated with pelvic fractures. ACS may also be secondary, such as from traumatic injuries to the extremities, septic shock, and severe burns. Risk factors include hypothermia, acidosis, and fluid resuscitation of greater than 5 L/24 hours. Symptoms include abdominal pain, dyspnea, dizziness, and weakness. Patient may exhibit distended abdomen, oliguria, hemodynamic instability, and respiratory distress. The most common measurement is intravesicular pressure in which a Foley catheter is inserted into the bladder and connected to an IV bag of NS with a pressure transducer in the line. The patient is placed in supine position and transducer leveled to the mid-axillary line. The bladder is filled with 1 mL/kg (to maximum of 25 mL) NS, then the tubing clamped. After 60 seconds, the mean pressure is obtained at the end of expiration.

MAXILLOFACIAL TRAUMA

Maxillofacial trauma is often accompanied by pain, swelling, bleeding, and bruising; the presence of one or more of these symptoms may indicate such trauma. Examine the teeth of the patient to determine if any have been knocked loose or knocked out. Examine the patient's jaw to uncover signs of dislocation. Assess upper respiratory functioning and look for signs of bruising around the eyes to help diagnose a fractured nose. Conduct an ocular examination to look for injuries to the eyes and the eye sockets. Blurred or double vision, limited eye mobility, and numbness in the ocular area may also be indicators of maxillofacial trauma of the eyes.

ASSESSING CRANIAL NERVE FUNCTIONING

A patient who presents with blindness in one (unilateral blindness) or both (bilateral blindness) eyes has likely sustained damage to his/her optic nerve, which is also known as cranial nerve II. Caused by direct ocular trauma, an injury to the oculomotor nerve – or cranial nerve III – may be characterized by a dilated, fixed pupil. The trochlear nerve – cranial nerve IV – may be injured if a patient has difficulty with inferior and medial eye movement. Patients who have difficulty moving their jaws and who have sharp, stabbing facial pain may have trigeminal nerve – cranial nerve V – damage. Damage to the facial nerve, which is known as cranial nerve VII, is often signified by facial paralysis; symptoms of facial paralysis include eyebrow droop, lack of ability to control tears, to close the eyes, and difficulty pursing lips.

OROPHARYNX

The oropharynx is located in the back of the mouth; it is part of the throat. It is the part of the pharynx that is connected to the oral cavity. As food enters the mouth, it passes through the oropharynx prior to reaching the esophagus. The oropharynx can provide important information that can lead to the detection of oral cancer. Signs of oral cancer can include mouth or lip sores that will not heal, a lump or lumps in the neck, red and white splotches on the throat or in the mouth, and/or experiencing difficult or painful swallowing. Abnormal growths in a patient's mouth and/or on a patient's tongue may also be signs of oral cancer.

PENETRATING NECK INJURY

Patients with a penetrating neck injury (such as a gunshot or knife wound) should be carefully screened to determine if they have cervical disc and/or spinal cord injuries. The airway should be immediately assessed, as the patient may require intubation and ventilation. Orotracheal intubation is most common. If the injury creates a tracheostomy site, this site can be intubated. Suctioning may be needed if blood is in the airway. Bleeding must be controlled with direct pressure and an occlusive dressing applied to venous injuries to prevent air emboli. General circulation must be assessed, as injury to great vessels may occur. If the wound is contaminated with debris, it should be irrigated with normal saline. If the patient is fully conscious and has no indications of spinal cord injury, spinal immobilization is not indicated. A rigid cervical color is usually not necessary unless there is neurological impairment.

EVALUATING MENTAL STATUS

When assessing a patient's mental status, note:

- Level of consciousness: AVPU assessment.
- Posture and behavior: Abnormal findings include restlessness, agitation, bizarre posturing, catatonia (immobility), and tics or other abnormal movements.
- Dress, grooming and hygiene: Kempt/unkempt, clean/dirty.
- Facial expressions: May vary widely (anxious, depressed, angry, sad, elated, fearful). Note whether expressions seem appropriate to situation/words.
- Speech/Language: Quantity, appropriate/inappropriate, rate, fluency. Note aphasia (inability to speak and/or understand words), dysphonia (abnormal voice/difficulty speaking), or dysarthria (difficulty speaking words).
- Mood: Nature and duration of current mood. Suicidal ideation.
- Thoughts/Perceptions: Note logic, relevance, and organization of thoughts and abnormal findings, such as thought blocking (sudden period of silence in the middle of sentence while speaking), flight of ideas (racing thoughts), incoherence, confabulation (producing distorted memories), loose association (responses not connected to questions or one sentence not connected to next), or transference (redirecting emotions to a substitute). Note homicidal or suicidal thoughts, obsessions, compulsions, delusions, illusions, and hallucinations.
- Judgment: Note insight, ability to make decisions, plan.

ALERT, LETHARGIC, AND OBTUNDED STAGES OF CONSCIOUSNESS

While there may be some motor skill deficiencies and/or confusion with an alert patient, he/she is still able to respond well to questions and is able to actively participate in a mental status examination. A lethargic patient generally displays characteristics of being drowsy; he/she may also appear to actually be asleep. While a lethargic patient may appear drowsy or asleep, he/she can be awakened relatively easily and can respond to questions in a reasonable manner. An obtunded patient is not awakened as easily as a lethargic patient, and he/she does not respond well to questions. The obtunded patient may participate in a mental status examination by responding to questions, but his/her responses tend to be difficult to understand, and the responses are typically not provided in the form of complete sentences.

TWO LEVELS OF THE UNCONSCIOUS STATE

The two levels of the unconscious state are stuporous and comatose. A stuporous patient is one who exhibits an extremely small degree of awareness without being able to communicate in a clear, appropriate manner. The stuporous patient often utters inappropriate words and/or moans in an incomprehensible fashion. A patient can either be in a light stuporous state or a deep stupor. A patient in a light stupor is generally able to respond to pain by moving his/her extremities in an attempt to protect against the source of the pain. However, a patient in a deep stupor typically does not display this protection response and often does not respond to pain at all. Coma is the ultimate state of unconsciousness in which a patient displays no signs of alertness. The comatose patient cannot be awakened with stimulation and does not respond to painful stimuli.

ASSESSMENT OF CRANIAL NERVES I, II, AND III

Cranial nerve I, the olfactory nerve, controls a person's sense of smell. Cranial nerve I can be evaluated by asking a patient to identify a familiar smell such as an orange. Cranial nerve II, the optic nerve, controls the visual field and sharpness of vision. Cranial nerve II can be evaluated by holding a certain number of fingers in front of a patient and asking him/her to identify the number of fingers. The optic nerve can also be assessed by moving an object along the patient's peripheral area and asking him/her to identify when the object comes into his/her line of vision. Cranial nerve III is the oculomotor nerve, which controls the pupil's reaction to stimuli. This nerve can be evaluated by shining a light in the patient's eye and observing the response of the pupil. A healthy, normal pupil will promptly constrict when it encounters direct light.

ASSESSMENT OF CRANIAL NERVES IV, V, AND VI

Cranial nerve IV, the trochlear nerve, is partially responsible for eye movement. Cranial nerve IV can be evaluated by asking a patient to follow another person's finger as it moves using only his/her eyes and not moving his/her head. Cranial nerve V, the trigeminal nerve, controls facial sensation and pain. Cranial nerve V can be evaluated by touching a patient's face to monitor for a response. Cranial nerve VI is the abducens nerve, which controls ocular motor function. This nerve can be evaluated by examining a patient's lateral eye movements.

ASSESSMENT OF CRANIAL NERVES VII, VIII, AND IX

Cranial nerve VII, the facial nerve, is responsible for motor functions in the patient's face. Cranial nerve VII can be evaluated by asking a patient to perform various facial movements and/or to make certain expressions. Cranial nerve VIII is the acoustic nerve; it is responsible for hearing and balance. The hearing component can be evaluated by making a noise such as a finger snap near a patient's ear and monitoring for a response. The balance component can be evaluated by performing Romberg's test. Romberg's test is conducted by having the patient stand with his/her eyes open, hands at his/her sides, and feet together; next, the patient stands in this position with his/her eyes closed for one minute to monitor whether he/she falls. Cranial nerve IX is the glossopharyngeal nerve, which controls swallowing and taste. This nerve can be evaluated by using a tongue depressor to test the patient's gag reflex.

ASSESSMENT OF CRANIAL NERVES X, XI, AND XII

Cranial nerve X, the vagus nerve, is partially responsible for tasks such as heart rate. Cranial nerve X can be evaluated by monitoring a patient's heart rate and/or his/her blood pressure, which may both be lowered if the vagus nerve is activated. Cranial nerve XI, the spinal accessory nerve, controls neck movement. Having a patient shrug his/her shoulders up and down is a good way to evaluate how cranial nerve XI is performing. Cranial nerve XII is the hypoglossal nerve, which controls tongue movements. The hypoglossal nerve can be evaluated by having a patient stick out his/her tongue and press against a tongue depressor to resist it; this provides an effective measure of tongue strength.

Gross Motor Skills

Gross motor skills are skills typically acquired during infancy and early childhood that involve an individual's large muscle groups; tasks involving gross motor skills typically require the patient's body to move in a coordinated manner. A number of activities can determine a patient's gross motor skills functioning; examples of such activities include walking, balancing on one leg, and jumping or hopping. Contrary to fine motor skills, gross motor skills do not decline when a patient is presented with a stressful situation; gross motor skill functioning has actually been found to improve when a patient encounters stress.

Fine Motor Skills

Fine motor skills are skills that generally require eye-hand coordination, as they are skills that involve smaller muscle groups. Activities that involve hand-eye coordination can help determine a patient's fine motor skills functioning; examples of such activities include having a patient pick up a small object in one hand and transfer the object to the opposite hand, writing a series of words on paper, and threading beads onto a string. Other activities that utilize a patient's smaller muscle groups and subsequently test his/her fine motor skills include whistling, making facial expressions, and articulating specific words.

Spinal Immobilization

To prevent interference with x-rays, jewelry should be removed from a patient prior to performing a spinal immobilization. Additionally, any sharp debris such as glass that is present on the patient should be removed as a means of preventing further injury. Once jewelry and sharp debris have been removed, the patient should be placed in a cervical collar; it is important that the patient's spine remain stabilized during this component of the immobilization procedure. When the cervical collar is in place, the patient should be transferred onto a backboard. As soon as the patient is centered on the backboard, blanket rolls or blocks should be placed so that the patient's spine is laterally stabilized. The patient's head should then be secured with straps to the board; finally, the patient's chest, hips, and knees should also be secured to the backboard with straps.

ICP Monitoring Devices

Intracranial pressure (ICP) is the pressure applied on the brain tissue, cerebrospinal fluid, and the blood circulating in the brain by the skull. In adult patients, signs of increased ICP can include vomiting; headaches; seizure activity; neurologic deficits such as an inability to speak, coordination difficulties, or changes in vision; behavioral changes; and/or a decrease in LOC. The intraventricular catheter may be used to monitor ICP and to drain excess CSF. CSF may be drained continuously or intermittently and must be monitored hourly for amount, color, and character. For ICP measurement, the patient's head must be elevated to 30 to 45° and the transducer leveled to the outer canthus of the eye. Normal ICP is 0-15 mm Hg on transducer or 80-180 mm H_2O on manometer. CFRNs should be familiar with ICP monitoring devices before interfacility transport. Never flush a device used for ICP monitoring, never used heparinized solution in the pressure tubing (only sterile NaCl), keep system free of air with tight connections, and use care when positioning patient to avoid decannulation. Be prepared to follow other orders to manage increases in ICP during transport including giving Mannitol, dexamethasone, draining CSF, and vasopressors for keep bp with a defined range. All orders should be reviewed before transporting this patient.

CEREBRAL EDEMA AND INCREASED INTRACRANIAL PRESSURE

Head injuries that occur at the time of trauma include fractures, contusions, hematomas, and diffuse cerebral and vascular injury. These injuries may result in hypoxia, increased intracranial pressure, and cerebral edema. Open injuries may result in infection. Patients often suffer initial hypertension, which increases intracranial pressure, decreasing perfusion. Often the primary problem with head trauma is a significant increase in swelling, which also interferes with perfusion, causing hypoxia and hypercapnia, which trigger increased blood flow. This increased volume at a time when injury impairs auto-regulation increases cerebral edema, which, in turn, increases intracranial pressure and results in a further decrease in perfusion with resultant ischemia. If pressure continues to rise, the brain may herniate. Concomitant hypotension may result in hypoventilation, further complicating treatment. During flight continuously monitor neurological status and vitals. Treatments include:

- Monitoring ICP and CCP
- Providing oxygen
- Elevating head of stretcher and maintaining body alignment
- Giving medications: Analgesics, anticonvulsants, and anesthetics
- Providing blood/fluids to stabilize hemodynamics
- Managing airway, providing mechanical ventilation if needed
- Providing osmotic agents, such as mannitol and hypertonic saline solution, to reduce cerebral edema.

HYPOXIC ENCEPHALOPATHY

Cerebral hypoxia (hypoxic encephalopathy) occurs when the oxygen supply to the brain is decreased. If hypoxia is mild, the brain compensates by increasing cerebral blood flow, but it can only double in volume and cannot compensate for severe hypoxic conditions. Hypoxia may be the result of insufficient oxygen in the environment, inadequate exchange at the alveolar level of the lungs, or inadequate circulation to the brain. Brain cells may begin dying within 5 minutes if deprived of adequate oxygenation, so any condition or trauma that interferes with oxygenation can result in brain damage:

- Near-drowning
- Asphyxia
- Cardiac arrest
- High altitude sickness
- Carbon monoxide
- Diseases that interfere with respiration, such as myasthenia gravis and amyotrophic lateral sclerosis
- Anesthesia complications

Symptoms include increasing neurological deficits, depending upon the degree and area of damage, with changes in mentation that range from confusion to coma. Prompt identification of the cause and increase in perfusion to the brain is critical for survival.

SAH

Subarachnoid hemorrhage (SAH) may occur after trauma but is common from rupture of a berry aneurysm or an arteriovenous malformation (AVM). However, there are a number of disorders that may be implicated: neoplasms, sickle cell disease, infection, hemophilia, and leukemia. The first presenting symptom may be complaints of severe headache, nausea and vomiting, nuchal rigidity, palsy related to cranial nerve compression, retinal hemorrhages, and papilledema. Late complications include hyponatremia and hydrocephalus. Symptoms worsen as intracranial pressure rises. SAH from aneurysm is classified as follows:

- Grade I: No symptoms or slight headache and nuchal rigidity.
- Grade II: Mod-severe headache with nuchal rigidity and cranial nerve palsy.
- Grade III: Drowsy, progressing to confusion or mild focal deficits.
- Grade IV: Stupor, with hemiparesis (mod-severe), early decerebrate rigidity, and vegetative disturbances.
- Grade V: Coma state with decerebrate rigidity.

Treatment includes:

- Identifying and treating underlying cause
- Observing for re-bleeding
- Anti-seizure medications (such as Dilantin®) to control seizures
- Antihypertensives
- Surgical repair if indicated

VENTRICULOSTOMY

A ventriculostomy involves placing a catheter in the ventricles of the brain. The catheter is attached to external tubing with a sampling port, a transducer (which must be leveled to the ear), a manometer, and drainage tub/bag in order to obtain the most accurate ICP measurements, allow for drainage of CSF (intermittently, not continuously) to control pressure, and to sample CSF. A ventriculostomy is required when there is obstruction in the brain, most often from bleeding or swelling that prevents adequate drainage of CSF, which is constantly produced at a rate of about 600 to 700 mL in 24 hours. The patient must be monitored continuously to ensure proper positioning, as sitting up during CSF drainage may result in rapid loss of CSF and damage to brain tissue. The drain must be clamped while the patient's position is changed. The CFRN must monitor pressure, drain CSF if pressure increases above baseline per protocol, monitor neurological signs, and assess insertion site and character of CSF for signs of infection.

EAR DRAINAGE

Inflammation or infection of some kind is one of the most common causes of ear drainage. Otitis externa, also known as swimmer's ear, is an inflammation that occurs in the ear canal or in the outer ear. The condition generally causes ear pain, itching or irritation, and ear drainage. Otitis media is an infection of the middle ear that can cause ear pain, a feeling of overall illness, vomiting, diarrhea, and/or hearing loss in the infected ear. Both otitis externa and otitis media are infections that can cause ear drainage. Certain things such as traumatic head injury, sudden changes in pressure, and extremely loud noises can rupture a patient's eardrum, which can also lead to ear drainage. Conditions that cause skin inflammation, such as eczema, can result in bleeding from the ear as well.

After a traumatic head injury, ear drainage that is suspected to be CSF can be tested quickly using the halo test, by placing a drop of the drainage on a filter paper. If the fluid creates a rapidly advancing halo ring it is most likely CSF, however this test can't differentiate between CSF and saliva.

CONDITIONS IN WHICH HYPERVENTILATION OF PATIENT WITH TRAUMATIC BRAIN INJURY IS INDICATED

While routine hyperventilation is not recommended as a first line of treatment in the majority of patients who have sustained traumatic brain injuries, there are instances with such patients in which hyperventilation may be indicated. Hyperventilation is indicated if the patient with a traumatic brain injury exhibits dilation in one or both pupils. Additionally, if the patient's pupils do not react in a balanced – or symmetric – manner, hyperventilation is likely indicated. It may also be indicated in patients who do not respond to pain and/or in patients who display other evidence of neurological deterioration.

CHEYNE-STOKES RESPIRATION

Often seen in patients who sustain significant head injuries, Cheyne-Stokes respiration is a pattern of abnormal breathing. The pattern is characterized by periods of shallow breathing alternating with periods of deep breathing. While the pattern involves a change in the volume of inspiration, the rate of respiration tends to remain fairly regular. Many patients who sustain significant head injuries develop increased intracranial pressure as well, and the Cheyne-Stokes pattern is frequently the first pattern of abnormal breathing to appear in such cases. The abnormal pattern is a result of a malfunction in the respiratory center of the brain.

GLASGOW COMA SCALE

The Glasgow coma scale (GCS) measures the depth and duration of coma or impaired level of consciousness and is used for post-operative assessment. The GCS measures three parameters: Best eye response, best verbal response, and best motor response, with a total possible score that ranges from 3 to 15:

Eye opening	4: Spontaneous. 3: To verbal stimuli. 2: To pain (not of face). 1: No response.
Verbal	5: Oriented. 4: Conversation confused, but can answer questions. 3: Uses inappropriate words. 2: Speech incomprehensible. 1: No response.
Motor	6: Moves on command. 5: Moves purposefully respond pain. 4: Withdraws in response to pain. 3: Decorticate posturing (flexion) in response to pain. 2: Decerebrate posturing (extension) in response to pain. 1: No response.

Injuries/conditions are classified according to the total score: 3-8 Coma; ≤ 8 Severe head injury; 9-12 Moderate head injury; 13-15 Mild head injury.

FRACTURES

The following are the nine types of fractures:

- Avulsion – fracture in which a tendon or ligament attached to a bone pulls off a fragment of the bone
- Comminuted – fracture in which the bone breaks, splinters, or fragments into more than one piece
- Compression – a fracture usually occurring in the spine whereby the bones are compressed or crushed
- Fracture dislocation – injury in which a fracture and a dislocation occur at the same time
- Greenstick – an incomplete break in which one side of a bone is broken and the other side of the bone is bent
- Impacted – fracture in which one of the fragment ends lodges into the other fragment end
- Oblique – fracture in which the break forms any angle other than a 90 degree angle with the axis of the bone
- Spiral – fracture produced by twisting a bone
- Transverse – fracture in which the break forms a 90 degree right angle with the axis of the bone

STABILIZING FOR TRANSPORT C1, C2, AND CERVICAL COMPRESSION FRACTURES

A patient is especially at risk for injury of the cervical spine in motor vehicle accidents that involve blunt impact with the windshield or ejection and high-speed motorcycle crashes as well as other types of direct facial, head, and neck injuries. If the patient has a suspected C1 or C2 injury or cervical compression fractures based on neurological assessment, a rigid cervical collar should be applied to limit motion. However, the cervical collar alone will not prevent flexion/extension movement, so it must be used in conjunction with a cervical immobilization device, which has restraining straps for the patient's forehead and chin. The cervical immobilization device is secured to a short or long spinal board. If the patient has difficulty breathing after cervical immobilization, the patient may require intubation and ventilation. If the patient is wearing a helmet and shoulder pads, they should be left in place until the patient arrives at the receiving facility unless they must be removed to secure the airway or better immobilize the head.

RIGID SPLINT, A SOFT SPLINT, AND A TRACTION SPLINT

A rigid splint may be constructed from material that is not easily pliable such as a piece of cardboard or a rolled newspaper. Rigid splints should be long enough to immobilize the entire fractured bone, they should be padded, and they should be anchored firmly to a non-injured body part. A rigid splint can generally be cut and formed to fit the extremity it is supporting. In contrast to a rigid splint, a soft splint is flexible. Examples of soft splints include pillows and folded towels or blankets. Despite its lack of rigidity, a soft splint has the capacity to provide adequate support to an injured body part when it is applied appropriately. Similar to a rigid splint, a traction splint does not bend easily. The purpose of a traction splint – unlike a rigid splint – is not to help correct a fracture but to immobilize the injured area during transport.

PRESERVING AMPUTATED BODY PART FOR SUCCESSFUL REIMPLANTATION

The first priority in caring for a patient with an amputated body part is to address life-threatening injuries and/or to resuscitate the patient. If possible, only one team member should handle the amputated body part to reduce the risk of contamination to exposed tissues. In all cases, the part should be handled with care. Tissue fragments from the amputated part should always be preserved – regardless of size – to assist with skin, bone, or nerve grafts that may be deemed necessary.

An amputated limb should be wrapped in saline soaked gauze or sealed in a plastic bag, labeled, and placed on top of ice in a container. It should not be washed unless it is contaminated with hazardous waste, and then proper protocols for decontamination must be followed. Care should be taken not to submerge the limb in ice water or cover with ice because this might result in freezing of the tissue and impairing its viability.

SHOULDER DISLOCATIONS

The two basic types of shoulder dislocations are anterior dislocation and posterior dislocation. An anterior dislocation is characterized by a bony protrusion in front of the patient's shoulder. Oftentimes, the arm of a patient with an anterior dislocation will be held away from the patient's body. Anterior dislocations are more common than posterior dislocations. Posterior dislocations are not as easily detected as anterior dislocations due to the fact that there is not typically an obvious physical deformity such as the bony protrusion common with the anterior variety. Patients with posterior shoulder dislocations generally hold their arms against their chest. Whenever possible, it is most effective to transport patients with anterior and posterior dislocations in a seated position.

COMPARTMENT SYNDROME

Compartment syndrome occurs when muscles, nerves, blood vessels, or bones within a confined space – a compartment – are squeezed together and have no place to expand. While it can occur in other areas, compartment syndrome occurs most often in the lower leg and forearm. Patients with compartment syndrome typically experience severe pain that does not respond to treatments including pain medication and/or elevation. Severe pain will result from moving a muscle running through the compartment and/or from squeezing the compartment. While severe pain in a centralized area is a key indicator of compartment syndrome, a test can definitively diagnose the condition. The test utilizes a needle attached to a pressure meter to determine the amount of pressure in the compartment. A pressure reading greater than 45 mmHg or within 30 mmHg of the diastolic blood pressure confirms the diagnosis of compartment syndrome.

SOFT TISSUE INJURIES

Soft tissue injuries can be caused by common, everyday activities. They are injuries that damage the ligaments, muscles, and/or tendons and include conditions such as sprains, strains, contusions, tendonitis, and bursitis. Sprains occur when ligaments are stretched or torn and are typically the result of a sudden twisting motion beyond the normal range of motion. Strains occur when a muscle is stretched or torn and are caused by overextending the muscle. Contusions can be identified by bruising around the injury site, as they occur when a blow is dealt to a ligament, muscle, and/or tendon. Tendonitis occurs when a tendon becomes inflamed; the inflammation causes severe pain or discomfort, particularly with movement. Bursitis occurs when areas surrounding the joints become inflamed from overuse. Tendonitis and bursitis often occur simultaneously.

FIRST, SECOND, AND THIRD DEGREE BURNS

A first degree burn typically only involves the outer layer of skin known as the epidermis and is characterized by redness and minor pain at the burn site. Second degree burns can be more painful at the burn site than first degree burns, but the level of pain associated with second degree burns depends on the amount of damage done to the nerves. Second degree burns generally cause the skin to blister and fill with fluid, as they frequently involve the papillary and reticular dermis, which

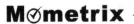

are layers of skin underneath the epidermis. Third degree burns are oftentimes characterized by a lack of pain, as the amount of nerve destruction involved with third degree burns is extensive. These types of burns often cause skin charring, they sometimes produce a purple fluid, and they can leave behind eschars, which are dead tissues that form over a burn wound like a scab.

RULE OF NINES METHOD TO ESTIMATE SIZE OF BURN WOUND

The *rule of nines* is a method utilized to determine what percent of an individual's total body mass is affected by a burn. The method is based on the notion that the human body can be divided into regions and assigned percentages that are multiples of nine percent. As a portion of total body surface area, the method allocates the following percentages to the adult body:

Region	Percent of body mass
Head	9%
Arm	9%
Arm	9%
Leg	18%
Leg	18%
Neck	1%
Chest and Abdomen	18%
Back and Buttocks	18%
TOTAL	100%

Using this method, if a patient is burned on both arms (18% total; 9% for each arm), the head (9%), the neck (1%), and the chest (18%), 46% of his/her body would be affected.

ESCHAROTOMY

Escharotomy is a procedure commonly used with burn patients. The purpose of performing such a procedure is to relieve pressure placed on the patient's tissue and to restore adequate circulation to the tissue. Eschar is the dead tissue that forms over a burn wound like a scab; oftentimes this scab interferes with a patient's circulation in his/her limbs, which can lead to limb loss. Without an escharotomy, respiratory complications can also develop. Escharotomy should be performed by making incisions – using sterile instruments – in the eschar to allow the tissue to break open, thereby releasing the pressure that was being placed on the tissue by the scabbing.

FLUID RESUSCITATION IN ADULT PATIENTS WITH BURN INJURIES

The primary purposes of fluid resuscitation in patients with burn injuries is to allow blood to flow to the tissues, to restore and/or maintain functioning to the vital organs, and to preserve tissue that has been damaged from the burn injury but remains viable. The patient's size and the severity of the burn injury are taken into account when calculating fluid resuscitation needs. The two most common formulas for calculating fluid resuscitation needs – the Parkland formula and the Modified Brooke formula – have been combined into the Consensus formula. This formula stipulates 2 to 4 ml/kg/%BSA where BSA represents body surface area. The first half of the fluids required should be delivered during the first eight hours following the injury, and the second half of the fluids should be administered within the 16 hours after those initial eight.

TREATING PATIENTS EXPOSED TO DANGEROUS SUBSTANCES

The patient who has been exposed to a dangerous substance should be moved to a location where the air is fresh and not contaminated. If oxygen is available, the patient should be supplied with oxygen. In cases where a patient is not breathing, cardiopulmonary resuscitation efforts should be initiated. If the patient's skin and/or eyes have been exposed to the dangerous substance, they should be flushed thoroughly with water. The flushing process should continue until it is evident that the dangerous substance no longer poses a threat to the patient's skin and/or eyes. Any clothing worn by the patient when he/she was exposed to the dangerous substance should be considered contaminated and should be properly removed and stored.

DECONTAMINATION PROCESS FOR PATIENTS EXPOSED TO HAZARDOUS MATERIALS

Patients exposed to a hazardous material should always be considered potentially contaminated. Any clothing the patient was wearing at the time of contamination should be removed in a designated location and stored there until disposal. Contaminated patients – and the flight personnel assisting the patient(s) – should be washed at least two times with water and/or water mixed with a mild soap. Personal protective equipment (PPE) worn by flight personnel during the decontamination process should also be removed and stored with the contaminated clothing. Anyone involved in the decontamination process – including the patient – should be evaluated for medical repercussions. Contaminated materials should be properly disposed of, and contaminated equipment should be decontaminated appropriately and thoroughly cleaned.

Any exposure/contamination should be reported at hand-off and to the appropriate infection control person, following protocols, and follow-up care should be sought if necessary. When reporting exposures/contamination, note the type of exposure, the date and time of exposure, circumstances, actions taken to decontaminate, and any other required information.

PATHOPHYSIOLOGY OF INHALATION INJURIES

There are three mechanisms by which inhalation injuries can occur. First, irritants can be inhaled and cause damage to cells as well as damage to the pulmonary parenchyma – the tissue of the lungs. Asphyxiants that deprive the body of oxygen can lead to hypoxemia, which is a second mechanism of inhalation injuries. Hypoxemia is a condition characterized by the blood not having an adequate supply of oxygen; its most common symptom is shortness of breath. The third mechanism by which inhalation injuries can occur is via absorption of a toxic substance into the bloodstream through the respiratory tract, which can lead to organ damage and/or organ failure, depending on the inhaled substance.

Special Populations

RUPTURED OVARIAN CYST

A patient with a ruptured ovarian cyst will likely experience pain when her abdomen is palpated. Additionally, when a pelvic examination is performed, a patient with a ruptured ovarian cyst will typically experience pain around her fallopian tubes and her ovaries. If severe hemorrhaging occurs in conjunction with the ruptured cyst, the patient will generally present with swelling in the abdominal area. For patients with severe hemorrhaging, orthostatic hypotension is a common finding upon physical examination. Patient should be placed in a position of comfort, assessed, monitored, IVs started and interventions for hypotension and shock initiated if needed during transport.

PREECLAMPSIA

Preeclampsia is a hypertensive disorder that occurs during pregnancy; the condition is characterized by the pregnant patient having high blood pressure and protein in the urine. Preeclampsia typically manifests late during the patient's second trimester of pregnancy or anytime during the third trimester. First-time mothers and mothers whose sister(s) and/or mother had the condition are more likely to develop preeclampsia. Additionally, patients who had high blood pressure or kidney disease prior to becoming pregnant are at an increased risk. Patients who are pregnant with multiple babies are also more likely to develop preeclampsia. The patient's age plays a role in determining her risk for the condition, as patients over 40 years of age and teenage patients have an increased risk of developing preeclampsia. As there is no cure, the only way to eliminate the condition is to deliver the baby via induction or caesarean section. However, if it is too early for the baby to live outside his/her mother's womb, delivery is not an option, and the condition must be managed via other means. Having the patient rest on her left side may help decrease her blood pressure, as it alleviates pressure from the patient's large blood vessels, thereby improving blood flow. Magnesium sulphate is sometimes administered intravenously to stabilize women with preeclampsia and to delay the onset of seizures in order to administer steroids that can help promote lung maturation in the baby.

ECLAMPSIA

Eclampsia is a condition characterized by convulsive seizures in pregnant patients. While many eclampsia seizures occur before, during, or after labor, it is possible to develop eclampsia as early as 20 weeks of pregnancy. Eclampsia is one of the leading causes of death for pregnant patients in the United States. The condition typically succeeds preeclampsia, a hypertensive disorder of pregnancy characterized by the pregnant patient having high blood pressure and protein in her urine; however, not all patients who develop preeclampsia will end up developing eclampsia. While eclampsia follows preeclampsia, symptoms of preeclampsia are not always noticeable in patients with eclampsia.

If the patient has altered mental status or seizures, secure and maintain airway. Even if the SpO2 reading is within normal limits the fetus may experience hypoxia due to vasoconstriction associated with preeclampsia, so give this patient oxygen unless contraindicated. Magnesium sulfate 4-6 grams over twenty minutes or maintenance magnesium infusion 1 to 2 grams/hour maybe ne used or prevent seizures or stop seizure activity. Magnesium sulfate also reduces vasoconstriction, providing the fetus with more blood and oxygen. If magnesium sulfate doesn't stop seizure activity, use benzodiazepines. Rapidly transport this patient to medical facility that handles OB emergencies.

PROLAPSED UMBILICAL CORD

A prolapsed umbilical cord is one in which the umbilical cord descends into the birth canal before the infant. This condition is extremely dangerous, as the infant can compress the cord during delivery, which would cut off his/her blood and oxygen supply. A prolapsed cord can lead to brain damage or death within minutes if it is not treated properly. The condition can also cause the infant's heart rate to decrease. Proper positioning of a patient with a prolapsed cord is crucial to the infant's survival. The best position for the patient is one in which pressure is taken off of the umbilical cord; examples of pressure-relieving positions include having the patient elevate her hips or having her get up on her hands and knees.

SEVERE VAGINAL BLEEDING

Severe vaginal bleeding can be characterized as bleeding directly from the vagina – not from a laceration or injury outside the vagina – that has the potential to soak more than eight super-size tampons or maxi pads in eight hours; severe vaginal bleeding can also be characterized by passing significantly-sized blood clots for a period of more than eight hours. Although vaginal bleeding is often difficult to control, pressure dressings should be applied to the site during transport. If an object in the vagina is the source of the bleeding, it should be left inside the vagina during transport. Severe vaginal bleeding that is accompanied by signs of shock, lower abdominal pain, fever, nausea and/or vomiting, and/or lightheadedness may be an indication of a serious complication or condition. In such cases, the flight team should make rapid transport to a facility that can handle gynecologic emergencies a priority in managing the condition.

CONSIDERATIONS FOR PREGNANT TRAUMA PATIENTS

Considerations for the pregnant trauma patient include:

- Spinal immobilization: Pregnant patients have impaired venous return when flat during the third trimester and increased risk of nausea and vomiting, so spinal immobilization should be used only with indications of neurological impairment. Once the patient is secured, the spinal board should be tilted 15-30° to the left (and head elevated if possible) to improve circulation to the placenta and avoid supine hypotensive syndrome.
- Hypoxia/Shock: With hypoxia, maternal blood is shunted from the fetal blood circulation to the mother's vital organs, and this can result in fetal distress, so it is critical to keep the mothers oxygen saturation level close to 100%.
- Cardiopulmonary resuscitation: Perform high quality chest compressions (2:30) as in non-pregnant patients and administer shock as soon as possible, administer 2 minutes of CPR between shocks

Prehospital: Administer 100% oxygen with non-rebreather mask at ≥15L/min. Use bag-mask ventilation with CPR. Insert two large-bore IV lines, infuse NS, and maintain continuous ECG monitoring.

UTERINE INVERSION

Uterine inversion occurs when the uterus turns inside out and protrudes through the cervix; in some cases, the top of the uterus comes out of the vagina. The condition is a potentially life-threatening one that can lead to severe hemorrhaging and shock. One way to manage uterine inversion is to attempt to manually return the uterus to its proper positioning; this attempt can be made by applying pressure to the top of the uterus with the fingertips and palm of the hand in order to push it back through the cervix. Once it has been repositioned, it is best to continue to apply pressure to the uterus with one hand inside the vagina and one hand on the patient's abdomen;

pressure should be applied in this manner until the uterus firms up. If the uterus is not easily put back in place, surgical intervention may be necessary.

PALPATING FOR UTERINE CONTRACTIONS

When a patient is having a contraction, it is typical for her entire abdominal area to tighten and feel hard. With the patient lying down, the examiner should place his/her fingertips on the uterus to palpate for contractions; the uterus will feel tight and hard when a contraction is occurring, and it should start to soften as the contraction comes to an end. Particularly near the end of a full-term pregnancy when a baby is larger in size, the patient's abdomen will feel hard where the baby's head and buttocks are located; however, this hardened feeling is not the same as a contraction, as the rest of the patient's abdominal area will remain soft if a contraction is not occurring.

TOCOLYTIC THERAPY

Tocolytic therapy is the use of medication to suppress the contractions of a patient in preterm labor, which is defined as labor that occurs before the 37th week of pregnancy. Tocolytic therapy should not be employed if the gestational age of the fetus is greater than 37 weeks or if the fetus weighs more than 2,500 grams. If the fetus is in acute distress, medication should not be administered to delay labor. If chorioamnionitis – inflammation of the membranes of the amniotic sac – is present, tocolytic therapy should not be employed. Additionally, if the patient has pregnancy-induced hypertension, eclampsia – a condition that causes convulsions, active vaginal bleeding, or cardiac disease, labor should be allowed to progress without introducing tocolytic therapy to suppress the patient's contractions.

BREECH PRESENTATION COMPLICATIONS

Complications with the umbilical cord are likely to occur with babies that present in a breech position; such complications include a prolapsed umbilical cord where the cord descends into the birth canal prior to the baby, a compressed umbilical cord whereby the baby's oxygen supply is compromised, and umbilical cord entanglement that can cut off the baby's oxygen supply and blood flow. Trauma and fractures may also be more likely to occur with babies in the breech position due to the potentially difficult and sometimes forceful deliveries they must undergo. Birth asphyxia – a condition characterized by an insufficient oxygen supply before, during or immediately after birth – is also more common in babies in the breech position than those who present in a head-down, vertex position.

EARLY DECELERATION, VARIABLE DECELERATION, AND LATE DECELERATION IN FHR

Early decelerations in a fetal heart rate (FHR) mimic the pattern of contraction; they tend to start at the beginning of a contraction and end when the contraction ends. This type of deceleration is harmless and is caused by head compression, which stimulates the vagus nerve. Early decelerations are most often seen when women are dilated between four and seven centimeters in active labor. Variable decelerations are caused by cord compression and can be seen at any time during the course of a contraction. They are characterized by a "V" or "W" shape on the fetal heart monitor. They are not typically associated with poor fetal outcome. Late decelerations generally begin after a contraction begins. After the onset of a late deceleration, the FHR gradually decelerates and then returns to baseline once the contraction ends. Late decelerations indicate that the baby is not receiving a sufficient amount of oxygen.

FETAL DISTRESS INTERVENTIONS

The patient should be placed in a left lateral recumbent position, which means she should be lying down on her left side. Placing the patient on her left side prevents compression of the inferior vena cava, which is a large vein that supplies blood to the heart from the lower half of the body; however, if placing the patient on her left side makes it difficult to provide appropriate care in the transport vehicle, it is acceptable to have her lie down on her right side. Using a mask, provide oxygen to the patient. Correct the problem(s) that led to the fetal distress if known. Keep monitoring the fetal heart rate (FHR), and follow appropriate protocols for abnormal FHR. IV fluids for the mother if there is questionable dehydration. Protect the umbilical cord from being compressed by the fetus's head if this is applicable and transport the patient to facility.

CONDITIONS THAT INCREASE RISK OF EMERGENCY DELIVERY

The labor and delivery process tends to progress more rapidly – consequently, the risk of an emergency delivery increases – when certain conditions exist. Patients who have given birth before – particularly those patients who have had a rapid delivery in the past – generally have faster deliveries with each successive pregnancy. Patients with certain connective tissue diseases, which are disorders involving abnormalities in the patient's collagen and elastin, are more likely to have fast deliveries. Pregnant women who have either sustained an injury and/or have been seriously ill during their pregnancy often have an increased risk of going into premature labor, which would necessitate an emergency delivery. Additionally, women with cervical incompetence, a condition whereby the cervix lacks the ability to stay closed when it should stay closed, generally have rapid deliveries.

RISK FOR DELIVERING DURING TRANSPORT

Several signs can help determine whether a pregnant patient may need to deliver her baby during transport. The patient should be considered to be in active labor if she is experiencing contractions in a regular pattern about three minutes apart that last approximately one minute each. If the patient is experiencing rectal pressure or a feeling similar to the urge to have a bowel movement, these sensations may indicate that the baby's head is in the birth canal and that the baby needs to be delivered. Additionally, if the flight team member can see the baby's head in the birth canal and/or if the birth canal appears to be bulging, the patient is at risk for delivering during transport. An uncontrollable desire to push is another strong indicator that delivery needs to occur promptly.

SHOULDER DYSTOCIA

Shoulder dystocia is a condition whereby a baby's shoulders are not able to progress through the birth canal after his/her head emerges. The condition oftentimes occurs with babies who are very large. Due to cord compression, time is a vital consideration in cases of shoulder dystocia; as such, delivery of the shoulders should be attempted prior to suctioning the baby's nose and mouth. Emptying a distended bladder may also be helpful. If an episiotomy incision has not already been made to enlarge the opening of the vagina for delivery, such an incision may assist in delivering the baby's shoulders. Performing the MC Roberts maneuver – a technique that involves flexing the patient's legs up towards her chest in order to increase the diameter of the pelvis – may also assist in delivery. Additionally, the application of suprapubic pressure in an attempt to manually dislodge one of the baby's shoulders can be an effective strategy for delivering the baby. If possible, and cord isn't being compressed or other emergencies are not present, rapid transport to a facility with OB emergency care.

UTERINE MASSAGE AFTER DELIVERY

Once the baby and the placenta have both been delivered, the fundus – or bottom – of the uterus should be manually massaged to aid with contraction. The uterine fundus should be massaged every 10 minutes during the first postpartum hour; the massage process can be repeated as many times as necessary during the second postpartum hour. After each massage session, the uterus should be palpated to ensure that it remains properly contracted and does not become relaxed and/or soft. Bleeding should also be assessed each time uterine massage is performed.

OPTIMAL SKIN, AXILLARY, AND RECTAL TEMPERATURE RANGES FOR NEWBORNS

The best temperature range for a newborn's skin is 36.0 degrees Celsius to 36.5 degrees Celsius. Optimal axillary and rectal temperature ranges for a newborn are 36.5 degrees Celsius to 37.0 degrees Celsius. The most important methods of heat loss in a newborn patient are convection and evaporation. Convection refers to heat loss resulting from air flowing over the patient's body. The cold temperature of a delivery room or of a flight transport vehicle can cause a newborn to lose heat through convection. Evaporation, whereby heat turns into vapor as it changes from a liquid to a gaseous state. Evaporation can cause heat loss in newborns, particularly if they are wet from fluids present during delivery and/or wet from being cleaned after delivery.

SUPPLYING OXYGEN TO NEONATES

A free-flow method of supplying oxygen near the baby's face may be used for a short period of time; however, this method is not ideal, as it is not possible to accurately measure how much oxygen the patient is actually receiving, and cold oxygen flowing onto the patient's face may also interfere with his/her thermoregulation. Hood oxygen allows flight team members to accurately measure how much oxygen the neonate is receiving, but it is difficult to have access to the patient's head without compromising the oxygen concentration when utilizing this method. Continuous positive airway pressure (CPAP) is another method of supplying oxygen to a neonate; CPAP can employ nasal prongs, a nasopharyngeal tube, or an endotracheal tube. While CPAP is an effective method of oxygen delivery, its drawback is the potential for having to perform an invasive intubation. Positive-pressure ventilation is another effective method, but it too requires intubation.

INDICATIONS THAT FETAL WELL-BEING MAY BE COMPROMISED

One indicator that fetal well-being may be compromised is the presence – over the course of several hours – of a substantial increase or decrease in the average, or baseline, fetal heart rate (FHR). An ideal baseline FHR should be between 120 and 160 for a period of 10 minutes; a baseline that "wanders" can also be an indicator that the well-being of the fetus is compromised. While fluctuations, or variability, in the FHR are normal and necessary, spontaneous decreases in variability or decreases that occur as labor advances may indicate a problem. Additionally, reduced variability accompanied by either bradycardia – abnormally slow heart rate – or tachycardia – abnormally fast heart rate – can also indicate a problem. Another indicator that fetal well-being may be compromised is the presence of subtle late decelerations, as they can be a sign that the baby is not receiving a sufficient amount of oxygen.

LACK OF RESPONSE TO NEONATAL RESUSCITATION

Mechanical problems, incorrect tube positioning, and unrecognized or undiagnosed medical problems are the most common reasons why infants do not respond properly to resuscitation efforts. Mechanical problems include such instances as not delivering an effective amount of oxygen to the infant or not providing an adequate amount of pressure during resuscitation attempts. In cases where intubation is necessary, the tube may be incorrectly inserted into a location other than the infant's trachea, which can also result in a lack of response to resuscitation efforts. When inserted properly, the infant's heart rate should immediately increase. A blocked tube can also present complications during resuscitation attempts. Other clinical or medical problems not directly related to the present problem may further complicate efforts to revive a neonatal patient.

GUIDELINES FOR NOT INITIATING OR DISCONTINUING RESUSCITATION EFFORTS IN NEONATAL PATIENTS

According to the American Academy of Pediatrics, circumstances may necessitate that resuscitation efforts with neonatal patients never be started or that they be stopped. The decision not to initiate resuscitation is usually made with the parents and a healthcare team. Resuscitation efforts may not be started if the patient weighs/weighed less than 400 grams at birth; they should also not be initiated if the patient's gestational age is less than 23 weeks. If the patient does not show any response to the resuscitation efforts for more than 10 minutes, they may be discontinued. Additionally, if the patient has a confirmed case of trisomy 13 or trisomy 18, efforts to resuscitate may not be initiated. Trisomy 13 and trisomy 18 are syndromes characterized by the presence of third chromosomes at chromosomes 13 and 18; the syndromes present multiple challenges to patients and make it difficult to survive more than a few months. Infants with congenital hydrocephalus – excess fluid around the brain – may also not be resuscitated. The CFRN should know laws relative to their state regarding neonatal resuscitation and be an advocate for the infant. Basic comforting care should be provided even if resuscitation isn't performed.

COMMON FEARS OF CHILDREN

For toddlers – one- to three-year-olds – a major fear is separation from their parents, guardians, or caretakers. At the toddler stage, fears about having their bodily orifices invaded begin to develop. Experiencing bodily injuries and/or pain are also common fears of toddlers. Additionally, toddlers fear losing control over objects in or aspects of their lives. At the preschool level – three- to five-year-olds – fears related to imaginary things such as monsters begin to surface as preschoolers' imaginations develop further. Fears about people such as kidnappers and robbers begin to develop as well at the preschool age as preschoolers become more aware of the world around them. Like toddlers, the fear of experiencing bodily injuries is common among preschool-age children. For school-age children – six- to 12-year-olds – common fears include experiencing bodily injuries, losing control over objects in or aspects of their lives, not being able to live up to others' expectations, and death.

ASSESSING CARDIOPULMONARY FUNCTIONING IN PEDIATRIC PATIENTS

Pediatric Advanced Life Support (PALS), is an assessment model that helps to quickly recognize and treat conditions that may be life threatening. First, a quick general assessment is done using the pediatric assessment triangle (PAT), which observes appearance, breathing and circulatory status. Appearance includes TICLS- tone, interactiveness, consolabilty, look, and speech/cry. Breathing notes obvious airway sounds, positioning used to aid breathing and accessory muscle use. Circulatory status is rapidly assessed by noting cyanosis or pallor. During this rapid assessment, obvious compromise can be recognized and treated. A child with an alteration in 2 to 3 of these areas is likely close to experiencing arrest. After this quick general assessment, the CFRN should rapidly assess airway, breathing, circulation, disability, and exposure.

The patient's airway is assessed initially and categorized as either: 1) clear, 2) able to be maintained once the patient is repositioned, or 3) not able to be maintained without intubation or removal of a foreign object. Next the child's breathing is assessed. Respiratory rate, effort, breath sounds, and skin color are all appropriate measures of the patient's ability or inability to breathe. To determine circulation, the patient's heart rate, pulse, blood pressure, level of alertness, skin color, and temperature are monitored. Disability uses the AVPU scale, GCS scale, and pupil response. Exposure assesses temperature, skin, and trauma evidence.

SAFETY PROCEDURES FOR TRANSPORTING PEDIATRIC PATIENTS WITH SPINAL INJURY

Steps must be taken when caring for a pediatric patient with spinal injury to ensure that the injury is not exacerbated. Cervical spine motion should be restricted, and movement of the patient's head and neck should be avoided, if possible. When assessing the patient's airway, the head should not be tilted per regular airway management protocol; rather, the patient's airway should be opened and maintained by thrusting the jaw. Due to the imperative nature of establishing an airway, the head-tilt maneuver may be utilized in situations where a jaw thrust is not feasible. Oftentimes, due to the disproportionate size of a child's head in relation to the rest of his/her body, the patient's torso must be elevated in order to prevent the transport backboard from imposing flexion on the cervical spine.

INFORMATION GATHERED THROUGH OBSERVATION OF AN INFANT

An infant in distress will likely show signs and symptoms of the distress even prior to a physical examination. An infant's nutritional state and fluid level can typically be observed without an examination as well. For example, an infant who looks emaciated may not be getting an adequate supply of calories, and an infant whose eyes look sunken may be insufficiently hydrated. The infant's overall shape can provide information about whether he/she may be suffering any injuries or has sustained any trauma. Skin tone and overall color can provide clues about the infant's temperature regulation and circulation. An infant's respiratory effort and his/her ability to cry may offer information about his/her airway and breathing. Additionally, the infant's posture provides indications of his/her gross motor skills functioning. Finally, the activity level and behavioral state of an infant can also provide information about the infant's state prior to a physical examination.

MORO AND STEP REFLEXES IN INFANTS

The Moro reflex can be tested by placing an infant in a supported position on a surface. With the examiner supporting the infant behind his/her neck with one hand and grasping the infant's hands with the other hand, the infant should feel relaxed and secure. When the infant's hands are suddenly released and the hand supporting his/her neck is relaxed, the infant should respond by throwing his/her arms outward. Additionally, an infant should clench his/her fists and look startled when the Moro reflex is tested. The Moro reflex tends to disappear around six months of age. The step reflex can be tested by supporting the infant under the arms and placing the soles of his/her feet on a surface; if the infant's step reflex is intact, he/she will making stepping motions even before the infant displays the ability to walk. The step reflex typically disappears by three months of age.

PALS PROCEDUREFOR BRADYCARDIA WITH A PULSE BUT POOR PERFUSION

In the pediatric patient with bradycardia (<60 bpm) and a pulse and signs of poor perfusion, attempt to identify cause. Signs of compromise include hypotension, sudden change in GCS, or signs of shock. Maintain airway, assist with ventilation as necessary, IV access, ECG, cardiac monitor and vital signs should be monitored. If this fixes the signs of poor perfusion, continue to observe will supporting ABC's and transporting for definitive care. However, if the heart rate remains less than 60 beats/minute with signs of cardiopulmonary compromise after implementing the above, start CPR. If bradycardia persists, epinephrine (0.01 mg/kg every 3-5 minutes IV) or atropine (0.02 mg/kg IV) can be given or pacing initiated. If the patient becomes pulseless, begin regular cardiac arrest protocol. If flight team personnel are able to determine causes for the patient's lack of responsiveness, attempts should be made to reverse those causes, if they are reversible.

PEDIATRIC TRAUMA SCORE

The Pediatric Trauma Score (PTS) is the most commonly used scoring method used in the assessment of pediatric trauma patients. A child with a score lower than 8 is at increased risk of morbidity, disability, and mortality.

Factor	+2	+1	-1
Weight	<20 kg	10-20 kg	<10 kg
Airway	Normal	Oral or nasal airway	Intubation or cricothyroidotomy
Systolic BP (mmHg) and pulse character	>90, good peripheral pulses	50-90, able to palpate carotid/femoral pulses.	<50, weak or absent pulses.
Level of consciousness	Awake	Obtunded, any loss of consciousness	Comatose
Cutaneous injury	No injury	Minor with contusion or laceration <7cm and not through fascia	Major with penetrating wound through fascia
Fractures	None	Single closed	Multiple open

ENDOTRACHEAL TUBE PLACEMENT IN PEDIATRIC PATIENTS

Specific considerations for ETT placement in pediatric patients include:

Some anatomy structures of children can make intubation and airway management in general more challenging. Their oropharyngeal structures are larger in comparison and their epiglottis tends to be large and floppy in nature. These anatomic structures can make intubation of children more difficult because visualizing the vocal chords is more challenging. Because the trachea is shorter, the ETT is more prone to be displaced. Children usually have a shorter time that they can tolerate apnea during RSI due to their decreased functional residual capacity and higher oxygen metabolism. They should be preoxygenated and monitored during RSI and provided bag mask ventilation as needed. As studies have proven that intubation success is higher with more training, and opportunities for intubation experience with pediatric patients is limited, providers should seek simulation training and other opportunities to gain experience. For a provider who does not feel that they have had sufficient experience, use of an LMA may be appropriate, as its placement is more likely to be correct in this situation.

POSSIBLE CAUSES FOR DETERIORATION IN INTUBATED PEDIATRIC PATIENTS

One of the most common causes for deterioration in the condition of an intubated pediatric patient is that the endotracheal tube has become dislodged or displaced from the patient's trachea. This can often be identified even before there is a change in a patient's condition as there will be a loss of end-tidal CO_2. Another common problem that can cause a patient's condition to worsen occurs when the tube becomes obstructed in some manner. Common causes of obstruction of the ETT include touching an internal mucosal surface, kinks in the tube, or secretions. It is also possible for equipment to fail while the patient is intubated, which would cause his/her condition to deteriorate. When a patient experiences a change in condition, equipment should be assessed and patient should be given oxygen by Ambu bag until the problem is identified and solved. Barotrauma, especially pneumothorax, which occurs when air or gas collects outside the patient's lungs, can also cause deterioration in his/her condition leading to a thoracostomy. Signs of pneumothorax can include shortness of breath, bluish skin tone, and an increased heart rate.

CARING FOR PEDIATRIC PATIENTS PRESENTING WITH PERSISTENT SYMPTOMATIC BRADYCARDIA WITH A PULSE

According to the Pediatric Advanced Life Support (PALS) bradycardia algorithm, the patient's airway, breathing, and circulation should be supported first, and oxygen should be administered. A defibrillator should then be set up and attached to the patient. If the patient's heart rate continues to remain lower than 60 beats per minute with poor perfusion, cardiopulmonary resuscitation (CPR) should be performed. If the patient is still showing signs of persistent symptomatic bradycardia, epinephrine should be administered through an intravenous line or an endotracheal tube every three to five minutes. A dose of atropine may be delivered if the patient's vagal tone is increased. Additionally, external cardiac pacing may be considered as an option to stimulate the heart and surrounding muscles to contract and help return the heart rate to normal range.

CPR FOR PEDIATRIC PATIENTS

For children between 1 and puberty, after assessing scene safety, if the patient is unresponsive, assess breathing while checking carotid pulse (only assess for 10 seconds). If there is no pulse, begin CPR. Do chest compressions using the heel of one hand in the center of the chest. One Rescuer: Begin cycles of 30 compressions and 2 breaths. Two Rescuers: Begin cycles of 15 compressions and 2 breaths. After the victim is connected to a defibrillator, check rhythm after 5 cycles (about 2 minutes) of CPR. If a defibrillator shows shockable rhythm, give shock and resume CPR immediately for two minutes. If possible, interruptions to the delivery of chest compressions should be minimized; flight team personnel should continue chest compressions after completing a rhythm check while the defibrillator is charging for another round of shock. Five cycles of CPR should be administered to the patient – lasting approximately two minutes – and then the patient's rhythm should be checked once again. Continue CPR and defibrillation until return of spontaneous circulation. For infants less than one, compressions may be either done with two fingers or with two thumb-encircling hands technique.

USING MANUAL DEFIBRILLATOR ON PEDIATRIC PATIENTS

When using a manual defibrillator on a pediatric patient, hand held paddles or adhesive electrode pads can be used, with electrode pads having more advantages. Electrode pads can be used to monitor heart rhythm, are not associated with sparks, have less chance of pad misplacement, and are safer for the rescuer. The electrodes should be as large as possible to fit on the patient's chest wall without having them touch. For pediatric patients who weigh more than 10 kilograms – typically children greater than one year of age – adult electrodes sized 12 centimeters are usually the most effective ones to use. For pediatric patients who weigh less than 10 kilograms – typically children less than one year of age – infant-sized electrodes are most effective during defibrillation. The pads may either be placed anterior/apex or anterior/posterior.

The first shock for a pediatric patient in ventricular fibrillation or pulseless ventricular tachycardia should be at 2 J/kg. When indicated, second shock should be at 4 J/kg and subsequent shocks at greater than equal to 4 J/kg with maximum energy 10 J/kg or the adult dosage.

Manual defibrillators are preferred but AEDs may be used when manual defibrillators are unavailable. If possible when using an AED for children less than 8 years old, use a pediatric dose attenuator system, however if this is not available use the AED without an attenuator for a shockable rhythm.

CONSIDERATIONS WHEN MANAGING PEDIATRIC SHOCK PATIENTS

One essential consideration when managing a pediatric shock patient is the patient's size. It is imperative to consider the patient's size when treating him/her to ensure that proper length-based resuscitation protocols are followed and that the right size equipment is used. Another consideration that needs to be made when working with a pediatric shock patient is the patient's increased risk for hypothermia and/or dehydration. Risks for such conditions are elevated in pediatric patients due to their immature systems and to the increase in their surface area to overall body mass ratio. While pediatric shock patients tend to experience a prolonged compensatory stage of shock, their state also tends to deteriorate faster than adults once they enter into the progressive stage.

SPECIAL CONSIDERATIONS FOR GERIATRIC PATIENTS

Geriatric patients have increased risk of injury and other morbidity because of the normal effects of aging as well as medications and chronic illness. Special considerations include:

- Dementia: Confusion may make patients combative and uncooperative. Patients may be unable to describe pain, so the PAINAD scale may be indicated. Some may require sedation for safe transport.
- Delirium: Older adults are prone to delirium with illness with sudden onset of fluctuating changes in consciousness with disorientation and confusion. Indications include the inability to spell first name backward or count backward from 20. Lorazepam, trazodone, or haloperidol may reduce symptoms.
- Falls: Older adults are especially at risk of falls, so mobility including the use of assistive devices should be assessed
- Skin tears/Bruising: Skin is more friable and may easily tear or bruise if grasped or pulled.
- Hypothermia: Because thermoregulation if often impaired, the older adult can experience hypothermia with environmental temperatures below 70° F, so the CFRN should avoid exposing the patient and should use warmed blankets to maintain temperature.

Geriatric patients are at risk of polypharmacy, the simultaneous use of many drugs, some of which may duplicate or interact with other drugs. Patients may have similar prescriptions from different physicians and may take multiple OTC drugs. Patients taking 5 different drugs have a 50% risk of interactions and 100% risk with 10 drugs. Additionally, aging affects pharmacokinetics:

- Absorption: While the percentage of drug absorbed changes little with age for most drugs, the rate of absorption slows, delaying response. Decreased gastric acidity may reduce absorption of some drugs.
- Distribution: Body water content, lean body mass, and protein binding sites decrease, and fat content increases, resulting in (1) increased storage of lipid-soluble drugs resulting in decreased plasma level and response, (2) decreased volume for water-soluble drugs resulting in intensified response, and (3) decreased protein binding resulting in increased free drug and intensified response.
- Metabolism: Decreased hepatic metabolism may result in increased half-life of drugs.
- Excretion: Decreased renal function may result in drug accumulation and adverse effects.

EFFICIENT AND ACCURATE PHYSICAL EXAMS ON BARIATRIC PATIENTS

The bariatric patient poses a number of physical examination challenges. Equipment must be appropriate for the patient's size to ensure correct results. For example, the inflatable bladder of a BP cuff should encircle at least 80% of the arm. If no adequate BP cuff is available, a thigh cuff may be substituted. Lung assessment should be done with auscultation on bare skin because of diminished breath sounds. Cardiovascular assessment should be done if possible with the patient leaning forward so the heart is in closer proximity to the chest wall, and the carotid pulse should be assessed along with the apical pulse. If the patient is supine, the patient should raise the arms above the head. Taking VS after exertion may result in elevated results, so patients should be allowed a few minutes rest first or VS should be reassessed. A tongue depressor may be necessary to view the posterior oropharynx. The liver scratch test may be utilized to assess the liver margin.

TRANSPORTING BARIATRIC PATIENTS

The first considerations when transporting bariatric patients are the ability to safely handle the patient and the availability of adequate personnel to facilitate transport. Transport equipment must be appropriate for the patient's size and weight (so it's important to ascertain the patient's weight), and the transport vehicle must be able to accommodate the patient. Some fixed-wing aircraft, for example, may have a door that is too narrow for patients weighing more than 400 pounds or steps that are difficult to maneuver. Loading through a cargo door (head first), if available, may be necessary. Loading ramps should be used to prevent injury to patient or personnel. Patients may require extra padding to prevent pressure during transport. Obese patients have increased risk of fat emboli and should receive 100% oxygen for at least 15 minutes before transport if possible. Patients may need light sedation if they experience claustrophobia because of the tight space in many aircraft.

AIRWAY MANAGEMENT AND DRUG DOSAGE CONSIDERATIONS FOR BARIATRIC PATIENTS

The bariatric patient is at increased risk of obstructive sleep apnea and hypoxemia when in supine position, so the patient should be transported with the head in semi-Fowler's position or upright to relieve pressure of the abdominal organs on the diaphragm if possible. Obesity makes it difficult to position the patient or to view the glottis for endotracheal intubation. Preoxygenation for 3 to 5 minutes before intubation per nasal cannula or non-invasive positive pressure ventilation may improve oxygenation. Two people should be used for bag-mask ventilation, which may be facilitated with insertion of an oropharyngeal or nasopharyngeal tube. The stacking maneuver (elevating the shoulders and head to raise the chin) rather than the sniffing position may facilitate ET intubation. When administering drugs based on ideal weight, the patient may receive inadequate medication, but administration based on actual weight may result in overdose, so weight is sometimes adjusted to 40% of actual weight minus ideal weight, but each medication should be checked in a drug-dosing reference table. If unsure, dosage is usually based on ideal weight.

CFRN Practice Test

1. Pulsus paradoxus is evaluated by:
   a. Heart rate (auscultation)
   b. Radial pulse (palpation)
   c. Systolic blood pressure readings
   d. Diastolic blood pressure readings

2. A patient involved in a car accident is being airlifted by helicopter over mountainous terrain more than 5000 feet above sea level. The patient is receiving intravenous (IV) fluids by gravity as the pump has malfunctioned. What effect will the increase in altitude to more than 5000 feet have on the IV infusion?
   a. There will be no effect
   b. The IV flow will stop
   c. The IV flow will increase
   d. The IV flow will decrease

3. A 17-year-old girl took an overdose of acetaminophen (thirty 500-mg tablets) in a suicide attempt; she told her parents, who called for emergency assistance, 8 hours after ingestion. Which of the following is the appropriate initial emergent treatment?
   a. N-acetylcysteine
   b. Gastrointestinal decontamination and instillation of activated charcoal
   c. Sodium bicarbonate
   d. Fomepizole

4. Which of the following arterial blood gas findings is consistent with metabolic acidosis in an adult?
   a. $HCO_3- < 22$ mEq/L and pH < 7.35
   b. $HCO_3- > 26$ mEq/L and pH > 7.45
   c. $PaCO_2$ 35–45 mm Hg and $PaO_2 \geq 80$ mg Hg
   d. $PaCO_2 > 55$ mm Hg and $PaO_2 < 60$ mg Hg

Questions 5 and 6 pertain to the following scenario:

A homeless man suffers a traumatic below-knee amputation and is awaiting airlift from a small rural hospital to a university hospital 200 miles away from the accident site for possible limb reattachment but becomes extremely confused and combative.

5. Which of the following is the most appropriate initial action?
   a. Arrange ground transport for the patient
   b. Provide physical restraints or chemical restraints
   c. Delay the flight until the patient calms
   d. Leave the patient at the rural hospital for treatment

6. What is the correct procedure for transporting the amputated limb?

    a. Submerge the amputated limb in ice water
    b. Place the amputated limb in a sealed plastic bag, label it, and submerge it in ice
    c. Clean the amputated limb with disinfectant to decontaminate it, and place it on ice
    d. Place the amputated limb in a sealed plastic bag, label it, and place it on top of ice

7. A tornado has caused significant damage in a rural town and multiple injuries. The closest hospital is 150 miles away. Only one helicopter is available for transport, but ambulances are scheduled to arrive within 15 minutes. After triage, which of the following patients should be airlifted?

    a. A 50-year-old woman with first- and second-degree burns on arms and hands (12% of body surface area)
    b. A 12-year-old boy with a fractured elbow
    c. A 25-year-old woman at 24 weeks' gestation in active labor
    d. A 45-year-old man with penetrating trauma in his left leg from shards of wood

8. Which of the following conditions is an absolute contraindication to nasotracheal intubation?

    a. Cervical spine injury
    b. Facial trauma
    c. Skull fracture
    d. Apnea

9. Using the "4-2-1" rule to determine maintenance fluid requirements, a child weighing 20 kg requires how much maintenance fluid per hour?

    a. 20 mL/hr
    b. 40 mL/hr
    c. 60 mL/hr
    d. 80 mL/hr

10. A patient with a traumatic head injury has the head elevated to 30 degrees and is receiving intravenous fluids and oxygen. During transport, the helicopter hits severe turbulence and incurs damage. The pilot tells the crew to prepare for a crash landing. Which is the correct action to prepare for the landing?

    a. Secure the patient in flat supine position
    b. Shut off the oxygen
    c. Remove the intravenous line
    d. Stand beside the patient to ensure his or her safety

11. All of the following patients are good candidates for air transfer by helicopter EXCEPT:

    a. A patient in active cardiac arrest with no improvement after 5 minutes of cardiopulmonary resuscitation
    b. A patient with burns covering 20% of the body
    c. An unconscious patient with a gunshot wound to the head
    d. A patient who has an acute stroke

12. What isolation procedures should be used to transport a patient with suspected active tuberculosis who is not receiving oxygen?

   a. High-efficiency particulate air (HEPA) respirators for the patient and staff
   b. Surgical masks for the patient and staff
   c. A non-rebreathing mask for the patient and HEPA respirators for the staff
   d. A surgical mask for the patient and HEPA respirators for the staff

13. A patient with acute abdominal pain arrived by hospital-owned ambulance at a private hospital. The triage nurse in the emergency department (ED) determined that he did not have insurance and insisted that he be immediately transferred to the county hospital 100 miles away rather than examined in the ED. The physician on staff refused to examine the patient. Both hospitals receive funds from Medicare. What should the flight nurse do when encountering this situation?

   a. Facilitate rapid transport to ensure the patient receives emergent care in accordance with regulations in the Emergency Medical Treatment and Active Labor Act (EMTALA)
   b. Refuse to accept the patient for transport because of EMTALA violations
   c. Accept the patient for transport, and report the triage nurse to the hospital administration
   d. Accept the patient for transport, and report the physician to the state medical practice board

14. A patient is being airlifted 500 miles by a high-altitude, fixed-wing aircraft. The patient has a Foley catheter and a cuffed endotracheal tube in place. Which of the following statements concerning this patient's condition is correct?

   a. The endotracheal cuff and Foley balloon should be inflated with air
   b. The endotracheal cuff and Foley balloon should be inflated with normal saline and monitored
   c. The endotracheal cuff and Foley balloon should be deflated and otherwise secured during transit
   d. High altitude has no affect on the endotracheal cuff or Foley balloon

15. A patient with severe facial and neck injuries cannot be successfully intubated but is in respiratory distress, so a needle cricothyrotomy must be performed. After the cricothyroid membrane is located and the trachea is stabilized, at which angle should the needle be inserted?

   a. 90 degrees
   b. 45 degrees rostrally
   c. 45 degrees caudally
   d. 60 degrees rostrally

16. The primary purpose of using rapid sequence intubation is to:

   a. Reduce the risk of gastric aspiration
   b. Prevent esophageal trauma
   c. Speed intubation
   d. Reduce tracheal trauma

17. A patient is to receive medication by intravenous (IV) line at the rate of 2 mg/min. The medication has a concentration of 10 mg/mL, and the IV tubing has a drop factor of 60. In this situation, the correct drip rate per minute is:

a. 6
b. 12
c. 20
d. 60

18. During transport in a helicopter or propeller aircraft, all of the following effects probably result from vibration EXCEPT:

a. Hypothermia
b. Fatigue
c. Abdominal pain
d. Impaired vision

19. An adult patient whose central venous pressure is monitored shows a falling pressure. Which procedure listed below confirms suspected hypovolemia?

a. Perform a rapid fluid infusion of 250–500 mL, and then evaluate in 10 minutes
b. Repeat readings every 5 minutes over 25 minutes to determine further decreases in pressure
c. Decrease rate of intravenous fluids, and observe for further decreases in pressure
d. Increase the rate of fluid infusion twice the current rate and evaluate for increases in pressure

20. Under the protocol of the American Council of Learned Societies for bradycardia with symptoms (i.e., shortness of breath, chest pain, hypotension), if an adult patient has no response to the first intravenous dose of 0.5 mg atropine, what should be done next?

a. Administer versed
b. Initiate transcutaneous pacing
c. Increase the next dose of atropine to 1 mg
d. Decrease the next dose of atropine to 0.2 mg

Questions 21–23 pertain to the following scenario:

A 7-year-old child was rescued from a burning home in which upholstered furniture, plastic toys, and a wool carpet caught fire. The child has black soot inside his mouth, his blood pressure is low, cardiac dysrhythmias are present, respirations are depressed, and he is faint and confused; he also experienced a seizure. He has burns over 15% of his body (i.e., the anterior surface of lower extremities and right palm) and a cut on his forehead.

21. Based on this history and the signs and symptoms, which of the following conditions are likely?

a. Cyanide toxicity
b. Carbon monoxide toxicity
c. Tracheal obstruction
d. Traumatic head injury

113

22. According to the Pediatric Advanced Life Support protocol and the presumptive diagnosis, which initial medication should be administered with rapid intravenous infusion?

    a. Albuterol aerosol
    b. Sodium thiosulfate
    c. Amyl nitrite
    d. Sodium nitrite

23. Based on the extent of the child's burns (15%) and his body weight (25 kg), using the Parkland formula (i.e., 4 mL X percent total body surface area burned X kg body weight), approximately how much intravenous fluid replacement does the child require in 24 hours?

    a. 0.5 L
    b. 1 L
    c. 1.5 L
    d. 2.0 L

24. A 17-year old man was bitten by a western diamondback rattlesnake on his right lower leg. The minimal indication for antivenin is:

    a. fang marks on the leg
    b. tenderness to palpation around the bite area
    c. patient insistence on receiving antivenin
    d. severe local pain and edema around the bite site

25. When unloading a patient from a helicopter, receiving medical personnel should be advised to:

    a. Immediately approach the helicopter from the front
    b. Wait until the helicopter shuts down (about 2 minutes)
    c. Approach the helicopter in a crouched position
    d. Approach the helicopter only when signaled to do so by the crew

26. During transit, a pregnant woman is about to deliver, but the umbilical cord is prolapsed. In what position should the woman be placed to relieve pressure on the cord?

    a. Supine
    b. Knees to chest
    c. Left lateral
    d. Right lateral

27. A 30-year old woman has second-degree frostbite of her feet with freezing extending into subcutaneous tissue, including muscles, tendons, and bones a with mottled appearance and non-blanching cyanosis, which will result in deep black eschar. Which of the following treatments is most appropriate initially?

    a. Wrap frostbitten areas in warm towels
    b. Massage frostbitten areas to stimulate circulation
    c. Begin slow rewarming with lukewarm water (26°C)
    d. Begin rapid rewarming with warm water (40–42°C)

28. A 60-year old man had symptoms of a myocardial infarction and suffered cardiac arrest but was resuscitated; he now has an irregular heart rate, pallor, and hypotension. The electrocardiogram (ECG) shows a 2 mm elevation of the ST segment in two contiguous leads with abnormal Q waves. All of the following are contraindications to fibrinolytic infusion EXCEPT:

    a. A history of stroke 6 weeks previously
    b. Anticoagulation therapy
    c. A history of craniotomy for removal of a neoplasm 4 weeks previously
    d. ECG findings

29. One hour after an emergency delivery of a term infant, palpation of the fundus shows that it is firm but deviates from the midline. The nurse suspects that the cause is:

    a. Uterine bleeding
    b. Bladder distention
    c. Normal variation
    d. Uterine rupture

30. A safe helicopter-landing site must include all of the following EXCEPT:

    a. A level surface area 60 x 60 to 100 X 100 feet
    b. An area cleared of debris
    c. An area free of power lines
    d. A level paved surface at least 60 X 60 feet

31. A patient has a transvenous pacemaker for drug-refractory dysrhythmia. What should the electrical output setting in milliamperes (mA), the maintenance threshold, be in relation to the stimulation threshold (ventricular pacing)?

    a. The mA should be one and a half to two times the stimulation threshold
    b. The mA should be one-half the stimulation threshold
    c. The mA should be three to four times the stimulation threshold
    d. The mA should equal the stimulation threshold

32. A pregnant woman has an emergency delivery at term. When evaluating the infant, what heart rate should be expected in the first 30 minutes after birth (first period of reactivity)?

    a. 160 beats/min
    b. 130 beats/min
    c. 100 beats/min
    d. 80 beats/min

33. The best position in which to place an older adult with heart failure to hear an S3 gallop rhythm is:

    a. Sitting upright
    b. Right lying
    c. Left lying
    d. Supine

34. The purpose of defusing sessions in critical incident stress management is to:
   a. Allow people to express feelings
   b. Provide a critique of the stress-inducing event
   c. Educate and provide guidance in handling feelings
   d. Identify signs of stress

35. A patient has chest pain, dyspnea, and hypotension. A 12-lead electrocardiogram shows atrial rates of 250 with regular ventricular rates of 100. P waves are saw-toothed (referred to as F waves), QRS shape and duration (0.4–0.11 seconds) is normal, PR interval is hard to calculate because of F waves, and the P: QRS ratio is 2–4:1. Which of the following diagnoses fits this profile?
   a. Premature atrial contraction
   b. Premature junctional contraction
   c. Atrial fibrillation
   d. Atrial flutter

36. A 44-year-old obese woman recovering from a femoropopliteal bypass develops sudden onset of dyspnea with chest pain on inspiration, cough, and fever of 39°C. A S4 gallop rhythm is present. The electrocardiogram shows tachycardia and nonspecific changes in ST and T waves. The most likely diagnosis is:
   a. Myocardial infarction
   b. Pulmonary embolism
   c. Pneumonia
   d. Sepsis.

37. A pregnant woman with mild contractions is evaluated for air transport. All of the following are signs of true labor EXCEPT:
   a. Bloody show
   b. Cervical dilatation
   c. Cervical effacement
   d. Regular rhythmic contractions

38. The correct procedure to evaluate the function of cranial nerve X (vagus) is to:
   a. Ask the patient to protrude the tongue and move it from side to side against a tongue depressor
   b. Observe the patient swallowing, and place sugar or salt on the back third of tongue to determine if the patient can differentiate the tastes
   c. Ask the patient to swallow and speak, and place a tongue blade on the posterior tongue or pharynx to elicit the gag reflex
   d. Place hands on the patient's shoulders, and ask the patient to shrug against resistance

39. A patient suffered cardiac trauma with tamponade and has an emergent unguided pericardiocentesis with electrocardiogram monitoring. As the needle is advanced and blood withdrawn, premature ventricular contractions occur. This most likely indicates:
   a. A normal response to the reduction in pressure
   b. An acute injury to the myocardium
   c. Laceration of the peritoneum
   d. Irritation of the epicardium

40. Before insertion of an intra-arterial balloon pump, the ankle–brachial index (ABI) is used to assess circulation of the lower extremities. If the brachial systolic pressure is 120 and the ankle systolic pressure is 90, what is the ABI?
    a. 0.75
    b. 1.3
    c. 30
    d. 210

41. When assessing capillary refill, a normal filling time is:
    a. < 0.5 second
    b. < 2 seconds
    c. 2–3 seconds
    d. 4 seconds

42. An infant died during an inter-hospital transfer; the sobbing mother takes the infant in her arms and refuses to relinquish the child. The most appropriate initial action is to:
    a. Provide the mother with a place to hold her child as long as she wants
    b. Ask family members to intervene
    c. Request that the hospital chaplain speak with the mother
    d. Explain the hospital procedures regarding death to the mother

43. In the Advanced Trauma Life Support protocol, during which step is a complete physical examination done on a trauma patient, including neurological assessment and defining a disability?
    a. Primary survey
    b. Resuscitation
    c. Secondary survey
    d. Definitive treatment

44. All of the following may interfere with the Glasgow coma scale assessment EXCEPT:
    a. Sedatives
    b. Facial edema
    c. Endotracheal intubation
    d. Intravenous fluids

45. The "death triangle" associated with rapid volume resuscitation and transfusions for treatment of hypovolemic shock include acidosis (metabolic), coagulopathy, and which of the following?
    a. Cerebral edema
    b. Hypothermia
    c. Increased hemorrhage
    d. Pulmonary edema

46. A 14-year-old child with brain trauma presents with status epilepticus and a series of tonic–clonic seizures with intervening time too short for the child to regain consciousness. Initial treatment should include:

    a. Rapid sequence intubation
    b. Acyclovir and ceftriaxone
    c. Phenytoin and phenobarbital
    d. Fast-acting benzodiazepine, such as lorazepam

47. A patient has a corneal abrasion from a soft contact lens. She complains of severe pain and intense photophobia. Initial treatment should include:

    a. Cycloplegic agent, such as cyclopentolate 1%
    b. An eye patch
    c. Erythromycin ophthalmic ointment
    d. Tobramycin ophthalmic ointment

48. An 18-kg child involved in a car accident has head and abdominal injuries and a pediatric trauma score of 5, which indicates which of the following conditions?

    a. Normal status
    b. Mild injury, requiring outpatient care only
    c. Major injury requiring admission to the critical care unit
    d. Impending death

49. An 8-year old African-American girl with sickle cell disease has developed pallor, tachycardia, weakness, and fatigue. She is recovering from a sore throat and has developed a "slapped face" rash, suggestive of parvovirus infection. What type of sickle cell crisis is most likely?

    a. Vaso-occlusive
    b. Aplastic
    c. Hemolytic
    d. Splenic sequestration

50. The minimal urinary output per hour expected for an adult patient is:

    a. 20 mL
    b. 30 mL
    c. 40 mL
    d. 50 mL

Answer Key and Explanations

1. C: Pulsus paradoxus is evaluated by systolic blood pressure readings. During the normal respiratory cycle, the blood pressure decreases slightly on inhalation while the pulse increases, and the blood pressure increases slightly on exhalation while the pulse decreases. This is exaggerated with pulsus paradoxus, which is evaluated by finding the first systolic reading during exhalation and then decreasing blood pressure cuff readings until the systolic pressure can be heard during both cycles. A difference between the exhalation-only systolic reading and the inhalation–exhalation reading of more than 10 mm Hg is positive for pulsus paradoxus.

2. C: The intravenous (IV) flow will increase, so adjustments to the flow rate may be necessary. Because barometric pressure affects the flow rate, a pump that adjusts to maintain a specified flow rate should be used whenever possible. As altitude increases, the barometric pressure decreases, and the reduced pressure allows flow to increase in the IV tubing. This may affect the dose of IV medications. For high-altitude fixed-wing air transports, cabins are pressurized but only to the equivalent of 6000–8000 feet, not to sea level.

3. A: N-acetylcysteine is the antidote for acetaminophen toxicity and is most effective in protecting the liver if given within 8 hours. Since 8 hours has elapsed in the case described in the question, the antidote should be given without waiting for serum levels as it decreases hepatotoxicity even if 24 hours have elapsed. Gastrointestinal decontamination is most effective if done within 1 hour of ingestion, although activated charcoal may have some protective effects if given within 4 hours of ingestion. Toxicity is plotted on the Rumack–Matthew nomogram with serum levels of more than 150 mg requiring an antidote. The 72-hour N-acetylcysteine protocol includes 140 mg/kg initially and 70 mg/kg every 4 hours for seventeen more doses (orally or intravenously).

4. A: Bicarbonate (HCO_3^-) less than 22 mEq/L and a pH less than 7.35 are consistent with metabolic acidosis, which may result from severe diarrhea, starvation, diabetic ketoacidosis, kidney failure, and aspirin toxicity. Symptoms may include headache, altered consciousness, and agitation to lethargy to coma. Cardiac dysrhythmias and Kussmaul respirations are common. The other readings listed in the question indicate the following:

- HCO_3 more than 26 mEq/L and a pH more than 7.45 are consistent with metabolic alkalosis
- $PaCO_2$ of 35–45 mm Hg and PaO_2 of 80 mg Hg or more are normal adult readings
- $PaCO_2$ more than 55 mm Hg and PaO_2 less than 60 mg Hg are consistent with acute respiratory failure in a previously healthy adult

5. B: Patients who are violent or combative should be physically restrained for transport and may also require chemical restraints to ensure personal safety as well as safety of the medical and flight crew. Because most rural hospitals lack the specialists and facilities needed to do limb reattachments, leaving the patient at the hospital is not a good option. Delaying transport by waiting or arranging ground transport may reduce the chance of successful reattachment.

6. D: An amputated limb should be sealed in a plastic bag, labeled, and placed on top of ice in a container. It should not be washed unless it is contaminated with hazardous waste, and then proper protocols for decontamination must be followed. Care should be taken not to submerge the limb in ice water or cover with ice because this might result in freezing of the tissue and impairing its viability.

7. C: A woman in active premature labor with a singleton or multiple births at 20 or more weeks' gestation should be airlifted because the infant or infants may be viable. Burns require air transport if they involve an explosion with respiratory distress or confusion, unconsciousness, or 18% or more (second- or third-degree burns) of body surface area is involved. Fractures can be immobilized for ground transport. Penetrating trauma (e.g., shrapnel, gunshot wound, stabbing) to the head, especially with prolonged unconsciousness, or trunk usually requires air transport, but injury to a limb, unless associated with severe bleeding or impaired circulation, is less critical.

8. D: Apnea is an absolute contraindication to nasotracheal intubation. The primary indications are suspected or confirmed cervical spine injury, resulting in a clenched jaw but with the gag reflex intact, and severe respiratory distress. Facial and skull fractures may, in some cases, be contraindications, depending on the location and extent of fractures. The nares size must be adequate to accept endotracheal tube in sizes 7 to 8. Usually a decongestant, such as phenylephrine, 0.5 mg, is administered to the nostril before tube insertion.

9. C: Maintenance fluid requirement for a 20-kg child is 60 mL/hr. The 4-2-1 rule is calculated by:

- 4 mL/kg/hr for first 10 kg
- 2 mL/kg/hr for second 10 kg
- 1 mL/kg/hr for remaining kg

Pediatric fluid deficits must be carefully estimated and managed. Fluid deficits should be replaced over 3 hours with half the first hour and a quarter in the remaining 2 hours. Fluid deficits are calculated by first finding the maintenance fluid requirement:

- Maintenance fluid mL X hours nothing by mouth = fluid deficit

10. B: The nurse should immediately shut off the oxygen because it may cause an explosion during a crash landing. Patients are usually positioned for impact with the head of the stretcher elevated to 30 degrees. Intravenous lines should be secured but remain in place. As with all takeoff and landings, medical staff and crew must be seated and secured by seatbelt. Helmets should be in place and secure. After crash landing, the crew should wait until the rotors stop turning to exit the aircraft and should meet at the nose of the aircraft or other safe place before attempting additional rescues if necessary.

11. A: A patient in active cardiac arrest is not a good candidate for air transfer because Federal Aviation Administration regulations require that all medical and flight staff be buckled in for safety during takeoff and landing, meaning that cardiopulmonary resuscitation (CPR) would be interrupted. Additionally, helicopters are usually staffed with two medical personnel and that may be inadequate to provide CPR and monitoring, and the likelihood that the patient could be resuscitated is low, so this is not a cost-effective use of air transport. Patients with burns over more than 18% of the body, gunshot wounds, or acute stroke are good candidates for air transport.

12. D: A patient with active tuberculosis should wear a surgical mask for transport, and the staff should wear high-efficiency particulate air (HEPA) respirators that are properly fitted and secured. A HEPA respirator should not be placed on the patient. A non-rebreathing mask is used if the patient requires oxygen (usually set at 10–15 L/min) during transportation. As with all patients, standard precautions, such as the use of gloves and eye protection to prevent contamination with blood or body fluids, should be used as well.

13. B: The flight nurse should refuse to accept the patient for transport as the hospital, which receives Medicare funds, has violated Emergency Medical Treatment and Active Labor Act regulations by failing to screen and stabilize the patient properly. Triage cannot be used instead of screening, which includes a physical examination, visual examination, history, and appropriate tests. Stabilization of the patient with emergency conditions or active labor must be done in the emergency department before transfer, and initial screening must be given before inquiring about insurance or ability to pay. Stabilization requires treatment for emergency conditions and reasonable belief that, although the emergency condition may not be completely resolved, the patient's condition will not deteriorate during transfer.

14. B: According to Boyle's law, at high altitude and decreased atmospheric pressure, gas volume expands, so an endotracheal tube or Foley catheter balloon filled with air may over-distend and burst; thus, normal saline should be used, especially for flights over 6000 feet although they must be monitored carefully as some expansion may still occur. This volume expansion may also affect injuries, such as pneumothorax. A tension pneumothorax may occur rapidly as altitude increases. Intracranial pressure may increase in those with open skull fractures as air becomes trapped and expands.

15. C: A needle cricothyrotomy is performed with the angiocath needle at 45 degrees caudally (aimed toward the feet). Prior to the insertion, the cricothyroid membrane is identified by palpating the thyroid cartilage and sliding the finger into the notch beneath. This space between the thyroid cartilage and the cricoid is the correct insertion site. The trachea must be stabilized between the thumb and fingers of one hand during the insertion. A popping sensation is felt as the needle enters the open space. Aspiration should show only air in the syringe. Blood or difficulty in aspiration may indicate incorrect placement. The needle is removed, and the catheter is advanced to the hub.

16. A: Rapid sequence intubation (RSI) is used to anesthetize and intubate the non-fasting patient to reduce risk of gastric aspiration. RSI may also be used for pregnant patients, very obese patients, and those with gastric reflux. Two intravenous lines should be in place before RSI and the patient preoxygenated for 3 minutes or more. Sellick's maneuver (pressure applied externally with thumb and index finger to the cricoid) is used to close off the esophagus and prevent aspiration. An induction agent (e.g., thiopental, diloxanide, propofol) is followed by a muscle relaxant (e.g., suxamethonium). Sixty seconds after the muscle relaxant, an endotracheal tube is inserted with a laryngoscopy, cuff inflated, secured, and placement verified by capnometer.

17. B: The drip rate should be 12 per minute based the following formula for a specific dosage:

- Dosage/min (2 mg) X drop factor (60)/concentration of drug/mL (10 mg/mL) = drip rate
- 2 X 60 = 120 divided by 10 = 12 drops/min

Drip rate for intravenous fluids per minute:

- The milliliters of infusion X drop factor/time in minutes = drip rate

Drip rate for medications prescribed based on dosage per weight in kg/min:

- Dosage per minute X kilogram X drop factor/concentration of drug/mL = drip rate

18. A: Hypothermia may result from temperature variations encountered at different locations and altitudes, but vibration may increase temperature as the body tries to cope with constant vibration. Other symptoms include fatigue related to stress, pain in the trunk (chest, abdomen), and impaired vision. Steps to reduce vibration include thick padding in seats and sitting with seat belts secured. Medical and flight crew should avoid touching or reclining against the walls of the aircraft as this increases the transmission of vibrations.

19. A: Because the most common reason for a fall in central venous pressure (CVP) is hypovolemia, a rapid fluid infusion of 250–500 mL may be given. If the pressure again starts to fall with 10 minutes or less, then the fall indicates probable hypovolemia. Serial readings should always be used to verify increases or decreases. CVP is the pressure in the superior vena cava near the right atrium and helps to evaluate the function of the right atrium and right ventricle and the flow of blood back into the heart. Normal ranges for CVP are 0–8 cm H2O or 2–6 mm Hg, depending on the type of measurement used.

20. B: Complete heart block may not respond to the first dose of atropine, so transcutaneous pacing should be initiated. With symptomatic bradycardia, after the airway is established, pulse oximetry, normal saline intravenously, and electrocardiographic monitoring, atropine is administered intravenously for adults at 0.5 mg push every 3–5 minutes (maximum 3 mg) and for children at the rate of 0.02 mg/kg push with a repeat in 5 minutes (minimum dose 0.1 mg). Versed may be given if necessary for sedation and comfort.

21. A: The symptoms experienced by the 7-year-old boy described in the question are consistent with cyanide toxicity, which should be suspected, especially when soot is found in the patient's mouth and low blood pressure and alterations in mental status are evident. Symptoms vary, according to the amount of exposure, but moderate-to-high inhaled concentrations may cause seizures and increasing cardiac dysrhythmias after initial tachycardia. Without prompt treatment, respiratory arrest, cardiovascular collapse, and death may occur. Cyanide is released from organic materials, such as wool, cotton, silk, wood, and paper, as well as plastics and polymers.

22. B: Sodium thiosulfate (400 mg/1.5 mL/kg to maximum of 12.5 g) should be given intravenously over 10 minutes because it binds directly to cyanide. Nitrites (found in some cyanide treatment kits) displace oxygen on the hemoglobin molecules, forming methemoglobin, thereby reducing the ability of hemoglobin to carry sufficient oxygen, and may result in unstable hemodynamic status. Albuterol aerosol (2.5 mg mixed in 2–3 mL normal saline) may be administered after sodium thiosulfate if respiratory distress (e.g., wheezing, decreased breath sounds, or extended exhalation) is present.

23. C: The Parkland formula is: 4 mL X kg body weight X body surface area (BSA). For this child described in the question, the equation is: 4 X 25 X 15 = 1500 mL or approximately 1.5 L per 24 hours. Fluids are usually replaced in the first 24 hours with half given in the first 8 hours after injury and the balance given over the remaining 16 hours. Electrolyte imbalances are most likely to occur with burns 20% of BSA. When calculating BSA of burns for children, each arm is 9%; each leg is 14%; head, back of torso, and front of torso are each 18%; and genitals are 1%.

24. D: Severe local pain and edema (signs of mild envenomation) around the bite site are indications for antivenin (5 vials). Because some bites are "dry" and antivenin is expensive, not readily available, and can have significant side effects, it is not given on request or without evidence of envenomation. Fang marks and some pain and local tenderness are common from trauma without envenomation. Moderate envenomation may include swelling beyond the area of bite, mild coagulopathy, and systemic manifestation with increasing symptoms with severe or life-threatening envenomation. Treatment may include 5–25 vials of antivenin, depending on the grade of envenomation and symptoms.

25. D: Patients should be unloaded only when a crewmember signals the receiving medical personnel to approach the aircraft. Prior to unloading, the crew usually shuts down the aircraft, and this requires about 2 minutes. A rotor aircraft, such as the helicopter, does not require that people approach in a crouched position, but people should avoid holding anything over their heads and should generally approach from the front of the aircraft and avoid the rear of the aircraft and the rear rotors.

26. B: Management of umbilical cord prolapse includes elevating the presenting part off the cord, having the mother elevate her knees to the chest, and preparing for C-section. A prolapse of the umbilical cord occurs when the umbilical cord precedes the fetus in the birth canal and becomes entrapped by the descending fetus. An occult cord prolapse occurs when the umbilical cord is beside or just ahead of the fetal head. About half of prolapses occur in the second stage of labor and relate to premature delivery, multiple gestation, polyhydramnios, breech delivery, and an excessively long umbilical cord.

27. D: Treatment for frostbite includes rapid rewarming with a warm water bath (40–42°C, 104–107.6°F) for 10–30 minutes or until the frostbitten area is erythematous and pliable as well as treatment for generalized hypothermia. After warming, treatment includes debridement of clear blisters but not hemorrhagic blisters. Frostbite most often affects the nose, ears, and distal extremities. As frostbite develops, the affected part feels numb and aches or throbs, becoming hard and insensate as the tissue freezes, resulting in circulatory impairment, necrosis of tissue, and gangrene. Three zones of injury include:

- Coagulation (usually distal): severe irreversible cellular damage
- Hyperemia (usually proximal): minimal cellular damage
- Stasis (between other two zones): severe but sometimes reversible damage

28. D: Fibrinolytic infusion is indicated for acute myocardial infarction (MI) under the following conditions:

- Symptoms of MI, less than 6–12 hours since the onset of symptoms
- 1 mm elevation or more of ST in two or more contiguous leads
- No contraindications and no cardiogenic shock

Fibrinolytic agents should be administered as soon as possible, within 30 minutes is best. All agents convert plasminogen to plasmin, which breaks down fibrin, dissolving clots:

- Streptokinase and anistreplase (first generation)
- Alteplase or tissue plasminogen activators (second generation)
- Reteplase and tenecteplase (third generation)

29. B: The fundus should be firm and midline. A deviation to one side or the other is often related to bladder distention, so this should be evaluated and the mother offered a bedpan or allowed to use a toilet if possible. If unable to urinate, she may need to be catheterized. Hemorrhage results in a boggy, soft fundus. Uterine rupture usually occurs during labor and is associated with pain, bleeding, and signs of shock.

30. D: A paved surface is not necessary for a helicopter-landing site, but level grassy or paved sites are preferred, ideally with 100 X 100 feet of clear space, but a minimum area of 60 X 60 feet may be used. Additionally, the area should be free of debris that may be disrupted by the rotor blades. The landing site should be clear of structures that may interfere with the aircraft, such as power poles, tall trees, power lines, cables, and antennas.

31. A: The electrical current in milliamperes (mA) delivers stimulation to the myocardium, and the setting for adequate ventricular pacing (the stimulation threshold) is determined in emergent situations by starting at a rate higher than the patient's intrinsic rate (usually about 20 mA) and decreasing until capture is lost and then increasing again until capture is regained. Once this setting is established, the maintenance threshold is usually set at one and a half to two times this level to prevent loss of capture with fluctuations in the stimulation threshold.

32. A: At term, the fetal heart rate usually ranges from 120–160 beats/min, and in the first period of reactivity (the first 30 minutes after birth), the heart rate is usually at the high end, about 160 beats/min. In the period of unresponsive sleep (30 minutes to 2 hours after birth), the heart rate usually drops to about 140 beats/min, and a heart murmur may be heard because of incomplete closure of the ductus arteriosus. In the second period of reactivity (2–6 hours after birth), the heart rate may become unstable and changing, varying between 120–160 beats/min.

33. C: S3 occurs after S2 in children and young adults and is a normal finding associated with rapid ventricular filling but may indicate heart failure or left ventricular failure in adults over 40 years of age; it is best auscultated with the patient lying on the left side and the stethoscope bell held firmly at the cardiac apex. S3 may also indicate mitral/tricuspid regurgitation that results in ventricular volume overload. The gallop sound occurs when the ventricle fails to eject all blood during systole so filling is impeded, causing a vibration.

34. C: Defusing sessions usually occur very early, sometimes during a stressful event, and are used to educate personnel about what to expect over the next few days and to provide guidance in handling feelings and stress. Debriefing sessions usually follow in 1–3 days and may be repeated periodically as needed. People are encouraged to express their feelings and emotions about the event. Critiquing the event or attempting to place blame is not productive as part of the Critical Incident Stress Management process.

35. D: Atrial flutter (AF) occurs when the atrial rate is faster (usually 250–400 beats/min) than the atrioventricular (AV) node conduction rate so not all of the beats are conducted into the ventricles (ventricular rate: 75–150 beats/min), as they are effectively blocked at the AV node, preventing ventricular fibrillation, although some extra ventricular impulses may go through. AF is caused by the same conditions that cause atrial fibrillation: coronary artery disease, valvular disease, pulmonary disease, heavy alcohol ingestion, and cardiac surgery. Treatment includes the following:

- Cardioversion if the condition is unstable
- Medications to slow ventricular rate and conduction through the AV node: diltiazem and verapamil
- Medications to convert to sinus rhythm: ibutilide fumarate injection, quinidine, disopyramide, and amiodarone

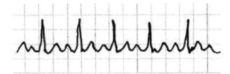

36. B: Although symptoms of pulmonary embolism may vary widely, depending on the size and location of the embolus, dyspnea, inspirational chest pain, cough, fever, S4 sounds, tachycardia, and nonspecific electrocardiogram changes in ST segments and T waves are common. Risk factors include obesity, recent surgery, history of deep vein thrombosis, and inactivity. Treatment includes oxygen, intravenous fluids, dobutamine for hypotension, analgesia for anxiety, and medications as indicated (digitalis, diuretic, antiarrhythmic). Intubation and mechanical ventilation may be required. A percutaneous filter may be placed in the inferior vena cava to prevent more emboli from reaching the lungs.

37. A: True labor may commence without bloody show, which is a bloody mucoid discharge that is often passed in the pre-labor period (usually about 24 hours prior to the beginning of labor). However, this does not occur in all women. The signs of true labor include:

- Cervical dilation (opening of the cervix): The cervix is dilated 4 cm or more
- Cervical effacement (thinning of the cervix): Usually 0% before labor, but early effacement is about 30%
- Regular rhythmic contractions: Early contractions have become more frequent (every 3–5 minutes, lasting 45–60 seconds)

38. C: To evaluate cranial nerve X (vagus), ask the patient to swallow and speak, observing for difficulty swallowing or hoarseness, and stimulate the back of the tongue or pharynx to elicit the gag reflex. Other examinations include:

- Cranial nerve IX (glossopharyngeal): Observe the patient swallowing, and place sugar or salt on the back third of tongue to determine if patient can differentiate between them.
- Cranial nerve XI (spinal accessory): Place hands on the patient's shoulders, and ask the patient to shrug against resistance.
- Cranial nerve XII (hypoglossal): Ask the patient to protrude the tongue and move it from side to side against a tongue depressor.

39. D: Premature ventricular contractions (PVCs) or increase in the amplitude of the T waves is consistent with irritation of the epicardium from contact with the needle, so the needle should be slowly withdrawn until the PVCs stop and the ECG returns to baseline readings. Acute injury to the myocardium may elicit changes in the ST segment or QRS complex. A laceration of the peritoneum may not be evident at the time of injury but may result in subsequent infection and peritonitis. Other injuries can include damage to coronary arteries or veins, pneumothorax, esophageal laceration, and pneumopericardium.

40. A: If the ankle systolic pressure is 90 and the brachial systolic pressure is 120, then 90/120 = 0.75. Ideally, the blood pressure at the ankle should be equal to that of the arm or slightly higher. The degree of disease relates to the score:

1.3: Abnormally high, may indicate calcification of vessel wall

- 1–1.1: Normal reading, asymptomatic
- < 0.95: Indicates narrowing of one or more leg blood vessels
- < 0.8: Moderate, often associated with intermittent claudication during exercise
- < 0.6–0.8: Borderline perfusion
- 0.5–0.75: Severe disease, ischemia
- < 0.5: Pain even at rest, limb threatened
- 0.25: Critical limb-threatening condition

41. B: Capillary refill time of 2 seconds or more may indicate shock with decreased tissue perfusion, dehydration, hypothermia, or peripheral vascular disease. Grasp the nail bed between the thumb and index finger and apply pressure for several seconds to cause blanching. Release the nail and count the seconds until the nail regains normal color. If checking the fingernail, elevate the hand above the heart after releasing pressure. If assessing the lower extremities, check both feet and more than one nail bed.

42. A: The mother should be provided a quiet space and allowed to hold the child. In this early stage of grief, the mother may be overwhelmed and barely able to comprehend what has happened. While the other actions may be appropriate at some point, asking the family members or chaplain to intervene before the mother has had time to begin the grieving process or listing hospital rules may just increase the mother's stress.

43. C: A complete physical examination is done as part of the secondary survey, including a neurological assessment. The Advanced Trauma Life Support protocol steps include:

- Primary survey: Assess the airway, breathing, and circulation (ABCs)
- Resuscitation: Actively resuscitate and stabilize the patient
- Secondary survey: Review the ABCs and add disability and exposure/examination to provide further information about the extent of injury
- Definitive treatment: Treat the patient, which may include surgery or other medical treatment

44. D: Intravenous fluids should not affect the Glasgow coma scale (GCS) assessment; however, sedatives may depress responses, and facial edema may make evaluation of eye responses difficult or impossible. Verbal responses are precluded with endotracheal intubation. When scoring, the nurse should document interfering factors. GCS measures the depth and duration of coma or impaired level of consciousness. The GCS measures three parameters: best eye response (1–4), best verbal response (1–5), and best motor response (1–6), with a total possible score that ranges from 3–15. Injuries/conditions are classified according to the total score: 3–8, coma; 8 or higher, severe head injury; 9–12, moderate head injury; and 13–15, mild head injury.

45. B: The "death triangle" associated with rapid resuscitation includes acidosis, coagulopathy, and hypothermia. Advanced Trauma Life Support protocol calls for 2 L (crystalloid) rapid bolus for adults and 20 mL/kg for children. Transfusions may be added with extensive blood loss. The protocol calls for two large bore intravenous (IV) lines, although a central line may be needed in some cases. Short tubing and compression may allow infusion rates up to 500 mL/min, but this may rapidly cool the patient. Hypothermia may increase coagulopathy, so warming IV fluids, keeping the ambient temperature at 21°C, and using warming blankets may help prevent complications.

46. D: The initial treatment for status epilepticus (SE) is a fast-acting benzodiazepine (e.g., lorazepam), often in steps with administration every 5 minutes until seizures subside. If there is no response to the first two doses of anticonvulsants (refractory SE), rapid sequence intubation (RSI), which involves sedation and paralytic anesthesia, may be done while therapy continues. Phenytoin and phenobarbital may be added, but combining phenobarbital and a benzodiazepine can cause apnea, so intubation may be necessary. Acyclovir and ceftriaxone may be administered if the cause is unknown as SE may be triggered by viral encephalitis.

47. A: The initial treatment for a corneal abrasion is a cycloplegic agent, such as cyclopentolate 1% to relieve pain and spasm. Corneal abrasion results from direct scratching or scraping trauma, causing a defect in the corneal epithelium. Infection with corneal ulceration can occur with abrasions. Organic sources of injury pose the danger of fungal infection, and soft contact lenses pose the danger of a Pseudomonas infection. If the corneal abrasion resulted from use of contact lenses, the eye should not be patched. Erythromycin ointment is used for injuries not related to contact lenses. Tobramycin ophthalmic ointment is used if injury is related to contact lens.

48. C: Pediatric trauma scores (PTS) 9–12 are within normal limits, but 8 or less indicates an increased risk of mortality and the need for critical care, with a score of 0 associated with 100% mortality. The PTS assesses with scores of +2, +1, and -1, with the individual scores totaled:

Child's weight (> 20 kg, 10–20 kg, < 10 kg)

Airway (normal, maintainable, not maintainable)

Blood pressure (systolic) or pulse (> 90 mm Hg, 50–90 mm Hg, or < 50 mm Hg)

Mental status (awake, obtunded, coma)

Bone injuries (closed, open, multiple fractures)

Skin injuries (none, minor, major or penetrating)

49. B: Parvovirus infection puts a child with sickle cell disease at risk for aplastic crisis because the virus decreases or stops production of red blood cells, so anemia worsens. A vaso-occlusive crisis, characterized by severe pain, occurs when sickled cells block microvasculature and cause hypoxia and tissue necrosis. Hemolytic crisis occurs with sudden increased destruction of red blood cells with severe drop in hemoglobin and hematocrit. Sequestration crisis occurs when blood pools in an encapsulated organ (e.g., spleen, liver), resulting in circulatory collapse. The organ may become enlarged and rupture.

50. B: The minimal urinary output for an adult patient is 30 mL/hr, although this level cannot be sustained for long periods, as a more normal output is 40–60 mL/hr. Minimal output for an infant or child is 0.5 mL/kg/hr. Output of less than 30 mL/0.5 mL may signal renal damage. Urinary output is influenced not only by renal status but also by hydration and medications. Vasoconstrictive medications may reduce urinary output. Patients may have low output after surgery and then diuresis as their systems clear anesthetic drugs and other medications.

How to Overcome Test Anxiety

Just the thought of taking a test is enough to make most people a little nervous. A test is an important event that can have a long-term impact on your future, so it's important to take it seriously and it's natural to feel anxious about performing well. But just because anxiety is normal, that doesn't mean that it's helpful in test taking, or that you should simply accept it as part of your life. Anxiety can have a variety of effects. These effects can be mild, like making you feel slightly nervous, or severe, like blocking your ability to focus or remember even a simple detail.

If you experience test anxiety—whether severe or mild—it's important to know how to beat it. To discover this, first you need to understand what causes test anxiety.

Causes of Test Anxiety

While we often think of anxiety as an uncontrollable emotional state, it can actually be caused by simple, practical things. One of the most common causes of test anxiety is that a person does not feel adequately prepared for their test. This feeling can be the result of many different issues such as poor study habits or lack of organization, but the most common culprit is time management. Starting to study too late, failing to organize your study time to cover all of the material, or being distracted while you study will mean that you're not well prepared for the test. This may lead to cramming the night before, which will cause you to be physically and mentally exhausted for the test. Poor time management also contributes to feelings of stress, fear, and hopelessness as you realize you are not well prepared but don't know what to do about it.

Other times, test anxiety is not related to your preparation for the test but comes from unresolved fear. This may be a past failure on a test, or poor performance on tests in general. It may come from comparing yourself to others who seem to be performing better or from the stress of living up to expectations. Anxiety may be driven by fears of the future—how failure on this test would affect your educational and career goals. These fears are often completely irrational, but they can still negatively impact your test performance.

> **Review Video: 3 Reasons You Have Test Anxiety**
> Visit mometrix.com/academy and enter code: 428468

128

Elements of Test Anxiety

As mentioned earlier, test anxiety is considered to be an emotional state, but it has physical and mental components as well. Sometimes you may not even realize that you are suffering from test anxiety until you notice the physical symptoms. These can include trembling hands, rapid heartbeat, sweating, nausea, and tense muscles. Extreme anxiety may lead to fainting or vomiting. Obviously, any of these symptoms can have a negative impact on testing. It is important to recognize them as soon as they begin to occur so that you can address the problem before it damages your performance.

> **Review Video: 3 Ways to Tell You Have Test Anxiety**
> Visit mometrix.com/academy and enter code: 927847

The mental components of test anxiety include trouble focusing and inability to remember learned information. During a test, your mind is on high alert, which can help you recall information and stay focused for an extended period of time. However, anxiety interferes with your mind's natural processes, causing you to blank out, even on the questions you know well. The strain of testing during anxiety makes it difficult to stay focused, especially on a test that may take several hours. Extreme anxiety can take a huge mental toll, making it difficult not only to recall test information but even to understand the test questions or pull your thoughts together.

> **Review Video: How Test Anxiety Affects Memory**
> Visit mometrix.com/academy and enter code: 609003

Effects of Test Anxiety

Test anxiety is like a disease—if left untreated, it will get progressively worse. Anxiety leads to poor performance, and this reinforces the feelings of fear and failure, which in turn lead to poor performances on subsequent tests. It can grow from a mild nervousness to a crippling condition. If allowed to progress, test anxiety can have a big impact on your schooling, and consequently on your future.

Test anxiety can spread to other parts of your life. Anxiety on tests can become anxiety in any stressful situation, and blanking on a test can turn into panicking in a job situation. But fortunately, you don't have to let anxiety rule your testing and determine your grades. There are a number of relatively simple steps you can take to move past anxiety and function normally on a test and in the rest of life.

> **Review Video: How Test Anxiety Impacts Your Grades**
> Visit mometrix.com/academy and enter code: 939819

Physical Steps for Beating Test Anxiety

While test anxiety is a serious problem, the good news is that it can be overcome. It doesn't have to control your ability to think and remember information. While it may take time, you can begin taking steps today to beat anxiety.

Just as your first hint that you may be struggling with anxiety comes from the physical symptoms, the first step to treating it is also physical. Rest is crucial for having a clear, strong mind. If you are tired, it is much easier to give in to anxiety. But if you establish good sleep habits, your body and mind will be ready to perform optimally, without the strain of exhaustion. Additionally, sleeping well helps you to retain information better, so you're more likely to recall the answers when you see the test questions.

Getting good sleep means more than going to bed on time. It's important to allow your brain time to relax. Take study breaks from time to time so it doesn't get overworked, and don't study right before bed. Take time to rest your mind before trying to rest your body, or you may find it difficult to fall asleep.

> **Review Video: The Importance of Sleep for Your Brain**
> Visit mometrix.com/academy and enter code: 319338

Along with sleep, other aspects of physical health are important in preparing for a test. Good nutrition is vital for good brain function. Sugary foods and drinks may give a burst of energy but this burst is followed by a crash, both physically and emotionally. Instead, fuel your body with protein and vitamin-rich foods.

Also, drink plenty of water. Dehydration can lead to headaches and exhaustion, especially if your brain is already under stress from the rigors of the test. Particularly if your test is a long one, drink water during the breaks. And if possible, take an energy-boosting snack to eat between sections.

> **Review Video: How Diet Can Affect your Mood**
> Visit mometrix.com/academy and enter code: 624317

Along with sleep and diet, a third important part of physical health is exercise. Maintaining a steady workout schedule is helpful, but even taking 5-minute study breaks to walk can help get your blood pumping faster and clear your head. Exercise also releases endorphins, which contribute to a positive feeling and can help combat test anxiety.

When you nurture your physical health, you are also contributing to your mental health. If your body is healthy, your mind is much more likely to be healthy as well. So take time to rest, nourish your body with healthy food and water, and get moving as much as possible. Taking these physical steps will make you stronger and more able to take the mental steps necessary to overcome test anxiety.

> **Review Video: How to Stay Healthy and Prevent Test Anxiety**
> Visit mometrix.com/academy and enter code: 877894

Mental Steps for Beating Test Anxiety

Working on the mental side of test anxiety can be more challenging, but as with the physical side, there are clear steps you can take to overcome it. As mentioned earlier, test anxiety often stems from lack of preparation, so the obvious solution is to prepare for the test. Effective studying may be the most important weapon you have for beating test anxiety, but you can and should employ several other mental tools to combat fear.

First, boost your confidence by reminding yourself of past success—tests or projects that you aced. If you're putting as much effort into preparing for this test as you did for those, there's no reason you should expect to fail here. Work hard to prepare; then trust your preparation.

Second, surround yourself with encouraging people. It can be helpful to find a study group, but be sure that the people you're around will encourage a positive attitude. If you spend time with others who are anxious or cynical, this will only contribute to your own anxiety. Look for others who are motivated to study hard from a desire to succeed, not from a fear of failure.

Third, reward yourself. A test is physically and mentally tiring, even without anxiety, and it can be helpful to have something to look forward to. Plan an activity following the test, regardless of the outcome, such as going to a movie or getting ice cream.

When you are taking the test, if you find yourself beginning to feel anxious, remind yourself that you know the material. Visualize successfully completing the test. Then take a few deep, relaxing breaths and return to it. Work through the questions carefully but with confidence, knowing that you are capable of succeeding.

Developing a healthy mental approach to test taking will also aid in other areas of life. Test anxiety affects more than just the actual test—it can be damaging to your mental health and even contribute to depression. It's important to beat test anxiety before it becomes a problem for more than testing.

> **Review Video: Test Anxiety and Depression**
> Visit mometrix.com/academy and enter code: 904704

Study Strategy

Being prepared for the test is necessary to combat anxiety, but what does being prepared look like? You may study for hours on end and still not feel prepared. What you need is a strategy for test prep. The next few pages outline our recommended steps to help you plan out and conquer the challenge of preparation.

STEP 1: SCOPE OUT THE TEST

Learn everything you can about the format (multiple choice, essay, etc.) and what will be on the test. Gather any study materials, course outlines, or sample exams that may be available. Not only will this help you to prepare, but knowing what to expect can help to alleviate test anxiety.

STEP 2: MAP OUT THE MATERIAL

Look through the textbook or study guide and make note of how many chapters or sections it has. Then divide these over the time you have. For example, if a book has 15 chapters and you have five days to study, you need to cover three chapters each day. Even better, if you have the time, leave an extra day at the end for overall review after you have gone through the material in depth.

If time is limited, you may need to prioritize the material. Look through it and make note of which sections you think you already have a good grasp on, and which need review. While you are studying, skim quickly through the familiar sections and take more time on the challenging parts. Write out your plan so you don't get lost as you go. Having a written plan also helps you feel more in control of the study, so anxiety is less likely to arise from feeling overwhelmed at the amount to cover.

STEP 3: GATHER YOUR TOOLS

Decide what study method works best for you. Do you prefer to highlight in the book as you study and then go back over the highlighted portions? Or do you type out notes of the important information? Or is it helpful to make flashcards that you can carry with you? Assemble the pens, index cards, highlighters, post-it notes, and any other materials you may need so you won't be distracted by getting up to find things while you study.

If you're having a hard time retaining the information or organizing your notes, experiment with different methods. For example, try color-coding by subject with colored pens, highlighters, or post-it notes. If you learn better by hearing, try recording yourself reading your notes so you can listen while in the car, working out, or simply sitting at your desk. Ask a friend to quiz you from your flashcards, or try teaching someone the material to solidify it in your mind.

STEP 4: CREATE YOUR ENVIRONMENT

It's important to avoid distractions while you study. This includes both the obvious distractions like visitors and the subtle distractions like an uncomfortable chair (or a too-comfortable couch that makes you want to fall asleep). Set up the best study environment possible: good lighting and a comfortable work area. If background music helps you focus, you may want to turn it on, but otherwise keep the room quiet. If you are using a computer to take notes, be sure you don't have any other windows open, especially applications like social media, games, or anything else that could distract you. Silence your phone and turn off notifications. Be sure to keep water close by so you stay hydrated while you study (but avoid unhealthy drinks and snacks).

Also, take into account the best time of day to study. Are you freshest first thing in the morning? Try to set aside some time then to work through the material. Is your mind clearer in the afternoon or evening? Schedule your study session then. Another method is to study at the same time of day that you will take the test, so that your brain gets used to working on the material at that time and will be ready to focus at test time.

STEP 5: STUDY!

Once you have done all the study preparation, it's time to settle into the actual studying. Sit down, take a few moments to settle your mind so you can focus, and begin to follow your study plan. Don't give in to distractions or let yourself procrastinate. This is your time to prepare so you'll be ready to fearlessly approach the test. Make the most of the time and stay focused.

Of course, you don't want to burn out. If you study too long you may find that you're not retaining the information very well. Take regular study breaks. For example, taking five minutes out of every hour to walk briskly, breathing deeply and swinging your arms, can help your mind stay fresh.

As you get to the end of each chapter or section, it's a good idea to do a quick review. Remind yourself of what you learned and work on any difficult parts. When you feel that you've mastered the material, move on to the next part. At the end of your study session, briefly skim through your notes again.

But while review is helpful, cramming last minute is NOT. If at all possible, work ahead so that you won't need to fit all your study into the last day. Cramming overloads your brain with more information than it can process and retain, and your tired mind may struggle to recall even previously learned information when it is overwhelmed with last-minute study. Also, the urgent nature of cramming and the stress placed on your brain contribute to anxiety. You'll be more likely to go to the test feeling unprepared and having trouble thinking clearly.

So don't cram, and don't stay up late before the test, even just to review your notes at a leisurely pace. Your brain needs rest more than it needs to go over the information again. In fact, plan to finish your studies by noon or early afternoon the day before the test. Give your brain the rest of the day to relax or focus on other things, and get a good night's sleep. Then you will be fresh for the test and better able to recall what you've studied.

STEP 6: TAKE A PRACTICE TEST

Many courses offer sample tests, either online or in the study materials. This is an excellent resource to check whether you have mastered the material, as well as to prepare for the test format and environment.

Check the test format ahead of time: the number of questions, the type (multiple choice, free response, etc.), and the time limit. Then create a plan for working through them. For example, if you have 30 minutes to take a 60-question test, your limit is 30 seconds per question. Spend less time on the questions you know well so that you can take more time on the difficult ones.

If you have time to take several practice tests, take the first one open book, with no time limit. Work through the questions at your own pace and make sure you fully understand them. Gradually work up to taking a test under test conditions: sit at a desk with all study materials put away and set a timer. Pace yourself to make sure you finish the test with time to spare and go back to check your answers if you have time.

After each test, check your answers. On the questions you missed, be sure you understand why you missed them. Did you misread the question (tests can use tricky wording)? Did you forget the information? Or was it something you hadn't learned? Go back and study any shaky areas that the practice tests reveal.

Taking these tests not only helps with your grade, but also aids in combating test anxiety. If you're already used to the test conditions, you're less likely to worry about it, and working through tests until you're scoring well gives you a confidence boost. Go through the practice tests until you feel comfortable, and then you can go into the test knowing that you're ready for it.

Test Tips

On test day, you should be confident, knowing that you've prepared well and are ready to answer the questions. But aside from preparation, there are several test day strategies you can employ to maximize your performance.

First, as stated before, get a good night's sleep the night before the test (and for several nights before that, if possible). Go into the test with a fresh, alert mind rather than staying up late to study.

Try not to change too much about your normal routine on the day of the test. It's important to eat a nutritious breakfast, but if you normally don't eat breakfast at all, consider eating just a protein bar. If you're a coffee drinker, go ahead and have your normal coffee. Just make sure you time it so that the caffeine doesn't wear off right in the middle of your test. Avoid sugary beverages, and drink enough water to stay hydrated but not so much that you need a restroom break 10 minutes into the test. If your test isn't first thing in the morning, consider going for a walk or doing a light workout before the test to get your blood flowing.

Allow yourself enough time to get ready, and leave for the test with plenty of time to spare so you won't have the anxiety of scrambling to arrive in time. Another reason to be early is to select a good seat. It's helpful to sit away from doors and windows, which can be distracting. Find a good seat, get out your supplies, and settle your mind before the test begins.

When the test begins, start by going over the instructions carefully, even if you already know what to expect. Make sure you avoid any careless mistakes by following the directions.

Then begin working through the questions, pacing yourself as you've practiced. If you're not sure on an answer, don't spend too much time on it, and don't let it shake your confidence. Either skip it and come back later, or eliminate as many wrong answers as possible and guess among the remaining ones. Don't dwell on these questions as you continue—put them out of your mind and focus on what lies ahead.

Be sure to read all of the answer choices, even if you're sure the first one is the right answer. Sometimes you'll find a better one if you keep reading. But don't second-guess yourself if you do immediately know the answer. Your gut instinct is usually right. Don't let test anxiety rob you of the information you know.

If you have time at the end of the test (and if the test format allows), go back and review your answers. Be cautious about changing any, since your first instinct tends to be correct, but make sure you didn't misread any of the questions or accidentally mark the wrong answer choice. Look over any you skipped and make an educated guess.

At the end, leave the test feeling confident. You've done your best, so don't waste time worrying about your performance or wishing you could change anything. Instead, celebrate the successful

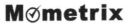

completion of this test. And finally, use this test to learn how to deal with anxiety even better next time.

> **Review Video: 5 Tips to Beat Test Anxiety**
> Visit mometrix.com/academy and enter code: 570656

Important Qualification

Not all anxiety is created equal. If your test anxiety is causing major issues in your life beyond the classroom or testing center, or if you are experiencing troubling physical symptoms related to your anxiety, it may be a sign of a serious physiological or psychological condition. If this sounds like your situation, we strongly encourage you to seek professional help.

Thank You

We at Mometrix would like to extend our heartfelt thanks to you, our friend and patron, for allowing us to play a part in your journey. It is a privilege to serve people from all walks of life who are unified in their commitment to building the best future they can for themselves.

The preparation you devote to these important testing milestones may be the most valuable educational opportunity you have for making a real difference in your life. We encourage you to put your heart into it—that feeling of succeeding, overcoming, and yes, conquering will be well worth the hours you've invested.

We want to hear your story, your struggles and your successes, and if you see any opportunities for us to improve our materials so we can help others even more effectively in the future, please share that with us as well. **The team at Mometrix would be absolutely thrilled to hear from you!** So please, send us an email (support@mometrix.com) and let's stay in touch.

> **If you'd like some additional help, check out these other resources we offer for your exam:**
> http://MometrixFlashcards.com/CFRN

Additional Bonus Material

Due to our efforts to try to keep this book to a manageable length, we've created a link that will give you access to all of your additional bonus material.

> Please visit https://www.mometrix.com/bonus948/cfrn to access the information.